Battered & Bruised But Not Out

Ronald Hixson

Bloomington, IN  Milton Keynes, UK

authorHOUSE™

AuthorHouse™
1663 Liberty Drive, Suite 200
Bloomington, IN 47403
www.authorhouse.com
Phone: 1-800-839-8640

AuthorHouse™ UK Ltd.
500 Avebury Boulevard
Central Milton Keynes, MK9 2BE
www.authorhouse.co.uk
Phone: 08001974150

First published by AuthorHouse 8/15/2006

ISBN: 1-4259-4236-9 (sc)

Library of Congress Control Number: 2006904879

Printed in the United States of America
Bloomington, Indiana

This book is printed on acid-free paper.

To Peggy
And
to those who passionately care about others and who continue to
be involved despite all the obstacles

Preface

This book was started because I felt stranded without a life line in a sea of confusion and constant danger. Attorney fees can be a good investment in helping you building a fence around your practice like the Internet's firewalls. As I wrote I began to discover how much more I needed to know and as I went from one fork in the road to another I soon found myself with so much information that my job turned more to rewriting, cut and pasting, and making choices of what to put in the book and what to leave out. Therefore, I don't see this book as a final word, only as a paragraph in a book of paragraphs.

As I wrote this book it occurred to me that there might be those who might read it as a book to run from private practice, that there are so many pitfalls to a private or small group practice that one might be better off becoming a plumber, electrician, teacher, or maybe a fisherman. There might be people reading this book who say that there are too many ways to lose your shirt, including going to jail, and not enough "rewards" and reasons to outweigh the negatives of practice. This is not all bad. This information can help you avoid some of the pitfalls and liabilities but not all of them. With this information you can better define your practice without having to learn "the hard way" and maybe save yourself 5 to 10 years of learning while practicing and perhaps save yourself thousands of dollars making the choice to structure your practice more defensively at the start-up and not 6 years later. In that case this book is clearly a bargain!

Ideas for this book come from those in practice, from Internet health care and news websites, from books about practicing without accepting managed care contracts, about economics of health care, financing health care, health care reform, policy decision making, and from personal experiences. It is a work in progress and is expected to change over the next few years as the discussion of public values and priorities push and pull on the national and state budgets. Those of us who stick our heads in the ground, denying all these signs, hoping that the storm of confusion passes over us without killing our practices, are likely to be out of business in the next few years if not sooner.

Our communities need the services of health care providers of all disciplines. No one group, i.e., surgeons, can operate alone. The body needs the mind and the head needs the body. We are interdependent providers which means that our survival depends on our adjusting to new trends and changes in political policies. We can adjust better if we work together across professional licensing and educational boundaries. The AMA has learned some hard lessons from their decisions to contract with MCOs and HMOs independent of any other health care provider. The unions have tried to unite different providers but unions, generally speaking, do not seem to understand ways and thinking of health care providers. It is therefore up to each health care provider to encourage their professional associations to work with professional associations of other disciplines. Instead of having 500,000 members then, we might reach three times that figure if we can just "all work together". Since politicians can understand the value of numbers, they can see the value of 1.5 to 2 million votes across the different states and what that might translate into financial support.

Working together to sell our "perspectives" of health care reform can attract more attention in political centers than a fragmented presentation. Becoming a part of the decision making process is seen as one answer to being pushed around by strange administrators and insensitive economists. People need to understand the value of what we do and how that translates into value in the economy. We need to change our thinking and language to be inclusive of business and economic terminology in order to connect with those sitting in policy chairs.

After reading this book you are encouraged to provide feedback either through my address or in the website that has been created to encourage providers to become activists for health care values. The website is www.practicenews.com.

Ronald Hixson, MBA, Ph.D. 2149 Del Rio Blvd., #103 Eagle Pass, TX 78852

Disclaimer

This information that follows is for your information, to use as you best see fit. It is not intended to be viewed as legal advice or as advice from a consultant or as an advice from a medical doctor. I am not now, nor have I ever been an attorney and it is not my intent to tell you what to do. At all times you should take information from here, as well as from other sources, and swing it by your legal team. You pay them a lot more than you will pay for this book. They are the ones who will represent you in court, not me. As I provide the following insights and information that I have obtained through the years of practice, I offer this to you so you can decide what pathway to follow. At no time should my advice be viewed as offering a guarantee or warrantee of any type that might confuse you into thinking that simply by reading my book you will know all the answers to all your questions and that no further check should be made. That could be a mistake. In all cases, any advice your attorney gives you should be followed before any advice I give.

Acknowledgements

This book is written as a challenge to those who have gotten so complacent that they no longer offer any resistance to the "establishment". Health care providers I have worked with or have some type of relationship with have unanimously agreed that we can no longer practice per our conscious (clinically and ethically) but from a defensive point of view (not just from being sued but being audited and threatened by insurance and state and federal investigators). Everyone seems to agree, "something needs to be done". This book is an attempt to get "something" started. I could not have written this book without having a supply of research available to me through the Internet and Amazon Books. Kaiser Family Foundation network is an extremely efficient and effective vehicle for gathering, storing, and sharing relevant health care information.

It took me over two years to research and build up the courage to venture into this new arena (book writing). I could not have done it without the great deal of encouragement from those that I care about and respect. Heather Blades edited my book, offering numerous suggestions and valuable ideas.

Those that have added their own level of support and encouragement have included Joe Pena, a school counselor in the Eagle Pass ISD, Hector Trevino, M.D., G. Surya, M.D., Elizabeth Alamillo, PA-C, Joe Heinz, PA-C, Richard Hood, M.D., Paul McCollum, Ph.D., Bob Schnoover, Ph.D., Curtis Cogburn, D.C., Carey Davis, D.C., Brent Fischer, MSW-ACP, and Jim Hunt, Vice President, Behavioral Health, Methodist Hospital, San Antonio. Herbert Garfield, M.D., has been immensely supportive, one of those "gold mines" found in a rural desert-like South Texas community.

Salvador J. Garcia, M.D. has been a rock of support, pointing me to areas of the community not being served and suggesting ways to both meet the mental health needs of a community while being able to pay the bills. Eliud Faz, M.D., has been a great resource of clinical skills and encouragements, helping me improve my diagnostic skills and understand the border communities and culture that you don't read about in books (yet). I appreciate the use of the library at Our Lady of the Lake University (OLLU), San Antonio, and to Joan Biever, Ph.D., Dean of Psychology, for her support of my research at OLLU Library. I am grateful to Dean Gilbert Bermea at Southwest Texas Junior College for his encouragement and for the use of the campus library for research. I want to acknowledge a special lady who was very instrumental during my assimilation and accommodation transitional phase setting up an office in Eagle Pass. Antonia Valdovinos is a wise lady who shares many of the concerns of this book and who offered a different perspective at times that was very useful.

Thanks to Pencye Hathaway who read my work and gave sound critiques, served on my non-profit organization's Board of Director and offered guidance on marketing strategies. Finally there is a special friend in Laredo who doesn't think I can do anything wrong and constantly asks about my book. "Uncle Ron, is your book done, yet?" To Megan: "I did it!" To Barney, my therapy dog, who taught me patience and a non-judgmental attitude, and who believes that there is more to life then work. You've earned another cookie, Barney.

Table of Contents

Part 1

WARNING! LANDMINES aHEAD

Choosing to be a health care provider may be hazardous to your
health, causing:

Bleeding ulcers
Excessive heart burn
Clogged arteries and gall stones
Chronic back, neck pain and loss of balance
Headaches, dizziness, nausea
Diverticulitis
Seizures, strokes and panic attacks
Confused thinking and foggy eyesight
Possible loss of hair and hearing
Dwindling savings account
Increased frustration and depression
More working hours and less "free" time
Sleepless nights and nightmares
Loss of credit and business
Loss of energy, joy and friends
Disillusionment
and
Possible death

Should you last five years in the practice of health care you will find
Some degrees of happiness and satisfaction,
You must reinforce your base of operation;
And you will find sources of rejuvenation,
Of relief, of inner peace.
Keep things in perspective, balance your time and your energy,
Never lose your sense of humor; hope is around the next bend in the
road.

And protect your Compassion with your mind and soul.

Chapter One
Shattered Glass

Summary

This chapter lays down a framework of basic issues by which all health care providers' practices will be influenced. It introduces the need for infrastructure, management techniques, and the danger inherent in liabilities and the financial risks of private practice. This chapter introduces the issue of public policy (how it is created and why) and why we should care. For those with thoughts of private practice, or development of a small group of multi-specialists, you will need this information BEFORE you incorporate so that you might be able to develop more realistic financial projections. For those that stay in academic or institutional organizations without entering practice, these issues can be obliging to one's quest for knowledge.

This chapter will help you do the following:

1. Readers will be able to name three reasons for studying business issues of a practice.
2. Readers will be able to apply some of the discussed concepts to their private or group practice.
3. Readers will be able to expand their awareness of how practitioners operate within a marketplace.
4. Readers will be able to change their perceptions of business and economic issues that affect the practice of health care.

Is Seeing Really Believing?

When you look into the mirror every morning, what do you see? A mother, father, son, daughter, grandparent, surgeon, a physical therapist or social worker, a nurse, maybe an entrepreneur or psychotherapist? The mirror doesn't say. What we see is what we want to see. A young slender beauty or an older quiet type? Sometimes we don't want to acknowledge what we see; sometimes the truth is uncomfortable. Some may even get mad enough to throw a hard object into the mirror, which shatters the glass. Picking up the pieces doesn't mean that anything has changed. In fact, it maybe even more upset because now you have an even bigger job, picking up all the pieces. When we consider new information sometimes are expectations, our dreams, may become shattered as much or more than the glass on the floor. After we clean up the glass, we must buy a new mirror.

When we consider new information, sometimes our expectations, our dreams, may become shattered. Our expectations and dreams are never the same, they have changed. We have changed. But we cannot fear having our expectations shattered. Instead we must do what we have to do – pick up the pieces and move forward! This book will help you realize truths about your work that may be difficult to see. At times you may feel frustrated, even angry, and want to "shatter the mirror". But remember that while your old ideas and dreams may be broken, you will be able to form new, more realistic dreams and expectations. And with this new knowledge you will have the tools to reach more goals, fulfilling more dreams. In the end, the image you will see a clearer reflection of reality, and it will empower you to make changes in your career.

It wasn't until Sigmund Freud wrote about his work that society took notice of this "new" form of practicing medicine. From then until now the practice of psychotherapy has grown in giant leaps at times, then steadily through fog of trial and error efforts, but always progressing with scientific and experiential documentation and creativity to where we stand today. In some ways, society has not kept up with the growth and development of psychotherapy services, such as issues of ethics, accessibility, financing, and infrastructure. This has caused a multitude of cognitive incongruencies within graduate programs as well as in the "field". For example, just because we can save a life with a transplant, do we want to pay for someone to have a transplant when that person has destroyed his mind and body with drugs? And do we want to offer marital therapy for couples who choose to beat each other up emotionally and physically? Other ethical questions that effect policies, health care financing and the direction of any standard of ethics include: Is society obligated to make health services available to those who choose to live along the border or in rural communities? And does everyone living in America have a "right" to health care at any cost?

The face of graduate training courses is changing even though traditionalists and purists resist any thing new. As far as the business side of health care, many professors don't have the academics or the experience to teach business, management and finance. Many have stayed gone from graduate school to the academic world forsaking the largest body of knowledge in world: experience. Undergraduate courses introduce the basics of psychology, the physical sciences. Graduate programs prepare students to tackle various clinical issues in depth but cover little about many of the legal, ethical, policies, and financing of health care which have a dramatic effect on any practice, private, group of multi-specialty. We (mental health disciplines) were taught tools of the trade: active and passive listening, psychological testing, mental status evaluations, documentation procedures, and setting boundaries, to name a few. However, few if any programs, offer more than as an elective course, one of the most important aspects of health care practice: the business side. (1)

Recently medical students are being taught how to communicate with their patients. This is being done because patients' complaints have increased about the lack of time with their doctor and they complain that doctors don't seem to listen to them after the first sentence. This type of approach to patient care has a way of encouraging doctor shopping and more lawsuits. Resident training programs have been viewed as spawning a bunch of egotistical self-centered geniuses. Medical schools have begun to respond to the emotional needs of the patient. In addition, as the last chapter will discuss, many of the future doctors are showing more political activism that was last seen in the 1960s as they push for a national health insurance because of the needs of patients. But it's also because they are realizing that foundations and employers can not be depended on to make up the difference between what the insurance policies pay and what the practice needs to meet payroll and office overhead expenses. If medical students can appreciate this need, why shouldn't mental health professionals, chiropractors, physical therapists, social workers and nurses also find ways to get involved in changing their professional training courses as well as getting more actively involved in the policymaking process?

The business part of a practice is more important than one piece of a puzzle that is missing. Each piece is important for the completion of a puzzle, but usually, a single piece will not stop one from seeing the entire picture. If you neglect the business side of therapy who may think you are creating a picture of a perfect practice when, in reality, you are creating a nightmare and possible financial ruin. Medical residents need to know the liabilities and costs of private practice. One of these is the treatment of joint pain. If everything has failed, the physician may choose to write a prescription for Kenalog injection. This injection costs the doctor $40. Medicaid reimburses the physician $1.40! This book will address not only the liabilities of practice but also the costs and the changing ethical face of practice. A look at the practice of health care will look different from the one you dreamed of during those warm summer college night, or when you started practice twenty years ago. Things are still changing, more wrinkles and bruises. Seeing and believing is enhanced when we are open to experience new ideas and entertain new directions.

I Get Dizzy When I'm in a Revolving Door

Over the past 100 years health care has changed in so many ways. As the 20th century grew so did the diversity of practitioners and with it controversy and charges of "extremism". There are still those who could be called social activists, while others might be said to be "out of touch" with the changing times. Others rebuke the "r" word (reform) because of how they interpret its meaning. In fact practitioners are often saying that having a traditional education in psychotherapy is a detriment and that they have to unlearn a lot of things that were taught in graduate school. Physicians are complaining that they are no longer in charge in the practice of health care. At one time everyone looked to the friendly family physician to bring their children into the world and to be with them and their parents at the end. The world of technology has sped-up the evolution of information and this has created certain liabilities and risks.

Managed care organizations (MCOs) are paid by states to manage the costs of health care. They are paid out of the pockets of providers. That is to say providers have lost anywhere from 20% to 60% of their reimbursement rates since MCOs took over. A majority of that reimbursement goes from providers to the MCOs. States are beginning to wake-up (though they still use MCOs) to the fact that MCOs are foxes who are placed to guard the chickens. However, in this case, the real farmer would never have done that. The present farmers (politicians) are much slower to learn the lessons that are taught in elementary school and so they still use the MCOs even though the MCOs have not saved any money. It was all a big joke! Everyone got it except the politicians who continue to support state contracts to MCOs. The pre-authorization process has become a time consuming process that costs the providers money. Even when pre-authorizations are given, some are taken back and payment denied. While this may not be as common in the general health care field as it is in workers' compensation cases, it is the providers who are being forced to work for "free".

Some cases are hindered by narrow restrictions of written health care policies. In one study the authors claimed that their reviews of preprogrammed medical charts of patients with anxiety disorders "revealed deterioration in some patients due to prolonged stays, compared with improved quality for misdiagnosed cases due to the intervention of the consulting psychiatrist during the program. These findings may prompt clinicians to question the impact of such programs on the patients' care. This legitimate concern is increasingly being addressed by managed-care firms' analyses of clinical outcomes. Although such clinical-outcome results are not yet systematically available, it is clear that managed care does extend the range of treatments available to patients when case managers are given the authority to override the narrow restrictions of written benefit plans and to certify a range of alternative treatments." (2)

Every time Medicaid changes MCOs there are inherent delays and interruptions in services, which translate into the provider paying for more services. When there is a Medicaid MCO change providers are not always told about it. They find out AFTER the change has been implemented and the previous MCOs begin to refuse pre-authorizations and reimbursements. Changes are coming so quickly and so close together it feels like you are in a revolving door and you can't get out very easily or safely. If the changes are coming too fast for the bureaucrats (governmental and MCOs) to handle properly, where is the logic for penalizing those who suffer the consequences? Is it any wonder why providers of every discipline are becoming increasingly hostile to both managed care organizations and the government? Another reason is that they feel raped by the greed of MCOs and the arrogance of the bureaucrats who operate from a level of leverage, not necessarily from any cognitive and rational basis. Raped in the sense that they are feeling abused, controlled, bullied, and have no reliable or easily assessable resource to fight back in a meaningful manner. "Raped" in terms of being held captive by an overwhelming force and not being able to resist or fend-off the attackers.

"From the point of view of physicians and other healthcare providers, the Health Insurance Portability and Accountability Act (HIPPA) of 1996, has been an unmitigated disaster. It has criminalized the practice of medicine, created fear and intimidation among healthcare providers and imposed unnecessary and onerous and administrative burdens upon them. Not only has HIPAA added to the costs and inefficiency of healthcare, but it also strikes at the very heart of the practice of medicine in the country – the doctor-patient relationship." (3)

The practice of health care is evolving and it is leaving the office and traveling to homes and schools and workplaces. It is active, brief, goal and solution orientated. It has become more open to the public and it has become more defensive. To survive in the wild and unpredictable political whirlpools that spring up frequently in every community, psychotherapists have had to spend more time managing their cases, their time, their costs, their resources. It is now not unusual to find a therapist calling one of their attorneys to discuss either a possible over-billing problem or maybe a professional liability issue. Or the therapist might call his/her attorney during patients to ask how to handle a subpoena, or a call from a HMO auditor or an investigator from the Attorney General's Office. The practice of health care has changed to a much more business orientation, more difficult to keep focused on client-centered issues and more stressful because of all the interference with limitations from new laws and contracts. In addition there are more demands but fewer revenues for an adequate infrastructure that is needed for much need protection from any allegations.

Providers are attempting to be creative in order to survive the rash of low reimbursement and the no-shows and re-scheduling problems. One way is to book 10 people every 15 or 20 minutes. This causes backups for obvious reasons, unless only one person shows up at that time. From the parents' point of view they complain about having to wait for long periods of time while the waiting room stacks up with sick families. One parent reported that she spends less time renewing her driver's license then waiting for her doctor. Another patient reported that he walked out after waiting two hours. The receptionist reported that "the doctor likes to spend time with his patients". If that is the case why not schedule more time between patients? Because people forget their appointment or because they find something else to do. The time allotted to a patient costs the provider money. Because reimbursement is so low, providers can not afford losing several hours a day to careless or thoughtless patients.

There are cases of walk-ins. Some physicians have simply given up on appointment scheduling and concentrated on walk-ins. Many people do not appear to appreciate the time it takes to see a patient, what the support staff has to do, what responsibilities and liabilities the doctor has and become very demanding of their time. There seems to be "you're here to serve me and my family. You're making all that money and you should be grateful for me coming to see you."

Some parents claim that their family doctor speeds through the exam and office, muttering, scribbling notes, and not really listening to what their concerns are. From the point of view of some doctors patients come in with one child then want to discuss another child which wasn't scheduled. Time is important to both patients and providers. Sometimes we, as providers, tend to forget the role of the family in the healing process because we do not have time to explain everything to them. Time is money, treating people takes time and energy. We catch their symptoms (physical and mental health) and often can spread it to other patients. Sometimes we just need to back off and re-examine what we are doing. Hopefully, this book will help in that regard.

This book is also written as an introduction to the discussion of the business side of therapy and health care which has gradually crowded clinical time with patients. The first goal of this book is to expand health care providers' awareness of the effects of certain costs and liabilities of health care practice. Secondly, it is presented to encourage health care graduate programs' Deans to add business courses to their graduate curriculums. Telling students that they can learn the business side of medicine or therapy "later" is like pushing your teenagers out the door when they turn 15 and say, "Now I've taught you everything I know. Go find a job and you'll learn what you need to know about life as you live it." Thirdly, it is hoped that this book will serve as a stimulus for political and social activism for change in our health care system.

Physicians practice differently then chiropractors, physical therapists and mental health therapists. We all have a common concern with the ethical practice of health care. Every health care discipline and license comes with legal and financial risks. We all need an infrastructure to help us survive but presently, with a change in political agendas and priorities, we no longer can afford the type of protection that hospital organizations and large group practices enjoy. The "other side" (in this adversary relationship, i.e. government agencies, HMOs and MCOs) has unlimited funds to find ways to investigate and prosecute health care professionals. Providers seldom if ever have any funds to defend themselves adequately.

Finally, therapists can use this book as a springboard to encourage more continuing education courses (on-line, professional seminars, and association conferences) that discuss those issues related to the business of developing a defensive practice; how to administrate, deliver and protect private or group practices. There is also the need to know more about the development of a marketing scheme that displays the VALUE of our services, not just list them in some order. We could also benefit from our professional associations have officers who become liaisons with other professional organizations for the purpose of setting a common good, promoting a common value, and fighting together in the legislative halls for our common values.

Spinning the Small Pie Slice Argument

While the standard economic analogy is a pie, perhaps a better one for our purposes is that of a cookie. When the pie is cooked there is a smaller expansion then when a cookie is baked and increases significantly in size. Therefore, when you slice a baked cookie, you get a larger slice then prior to being cooked. Being cooked is an analogy to the business of therapy as is the place of health care to the marketplace. When the economy is expanding and growing then you will have larger costs for healthcare but people will get more services for their dollars. This is another point to the issue of value and worth. We know that our services have value, but we often lack the ability to communicate this worth because we lack the hard data to support our claims. Thirdly, we have done a very poor job in educating the policy makers and the politicians.

Is it as simple as baking more cookies? What happens when we run out of dough? One argument may be that we can tax people and pay for anything they need, perhaps like Germany and Canada. Taxes are about 50% anyway when you consider tax on consumption. And we still lack access to the "best health care that money can buy". If we choose not to purchase health care insurance, then the issue of limited resources is something that can not go unanswered. The financing of health care is currently dependent on "sharing the risks". If people can not or do not purchase insurance policies then they apply greater burden on others sources, i.e., their neighbors' who now most pay more taxes to reimburse hospitals for indigent care. If we, as a society, say no new taxes, then are we willing to say there is a limit on what health care services might be available to the consumer or just to a certain population? Any limitation of health care smacks of rationing, which is what managed care organizations get blamed for today.

Even if we had all the money in the world, the infrastructure, for the administration and delivery of health care, is lacking and would costs millions to build. AIDS, or any other disease or disorder that is chronic, demands development of advanced health infrastructure. If we use the lack of infrastructure as an excuse to stop us from treating the sick and building the needed infrastructure, it is a circular argument. Now the lack of infrastructure AND the lack of will to build one are keeping adequate physical and mental health care from all the people who need it. Included within the infrastructure is adequate number of professional and those with appropriate training and skills. Without adequate funding and infrastructure it's very difficult to entice adequate professionals to the communities needing them. Therefore, we are reducing accessibility and denying adequate health care for populations that do not live in areas (mainly metropolitan communities) where there is sufficient health care services and professionals. While cookie dough will expand with baking, without baking there is no expansion. If infrastructure is not "worth it" why does the government have it? Why do the state legislators allow MCOs and health maintenance organizations (HMOs) to bill the states for layers of infrastructure and training in their organizations' programs? The states all these organizations to be created to go after that 25% to 30% that are taken away from providers so MCOs and HMOs can administer Medicaid and Medicare for the government. The MCOs and HMOs have sent layers of lobbyists to sell their programs and promising to save the state millions of dollars. Lobbyists have been a long time but in recent years companies have spent much more money getting their causes funded, approved or another project voted down. During last year's session ATT spent between $4 − $7 million for 112 lobbyists to push their cause (the deregulation of the phone giant). Todd Baxter, a cable-industry lobbyist who served in the Texas House during the 2005 session provides some insight in the lobbyist-legislator relationship that influences votes, laws, and funded programs. "There's no doubt that the number of lobbyists hired and the caliber of lobbyists they've hired have played a big role in their legislative wins. They certainly spend a lot, but from their perspective, they stand to gain a lot when their successful." (4)

"Learning to live and work within the ambiguities of the profession (health care) presents a challenge and an opportunity for the independent practitioner. We have witnessed the growth and placement of alphabet soup organizations (MCOs, HMOs, PPOs and EAPs, etc.) designed to contain costs and provide management for healthcare providers." (5) PPOs (preferred provider organizations) are groups of providers who contract as a group with MCOs and HMOs and are paid on a fee-for-service basis which usually means at a lower rate then their normal service fees. With increases of liability costs, rising administrative and overhead costs and lower reimbursements, those who remain or choose private practice will need to be knowledgeable about both health care and running a business. The opportunities in private practice will be less but still available. "The opportunities most likely will be there for those who are willing to conceive creatively of themselves as both therapists (and health care provider) and businesspeople. Those in private practice will need to accept the fact that what they do is both a service and a business" (6)   Health care services are a product that needs to be marketed and promoted for its value to the population served not just viewed as an expense.

Conflict with Values

People will ask why the system of health care is larger now than it once was years ago. Historians may respond that in 1950 the medical system was very small. Secondly, economists report a comparison between yesterday's dollars and today's, for example, that health care dollars equaled $1 for every $25 spent in the marketplace in the 1950s. Today they report that its $1 for every $7, maybe $6. Some project that it won't be long before it reaches $1 in $3. If you think about, what did we spend for groceries in the 50s? For gasoline? Housing? Much less then today. When you compare it to the percentage of your income, then you may be surprised to find that the percentages are less then you think, except for gasoline, and if you live in California perhaps housing. The issue isn't just about total costs, since there are more people living in the United States now then in 1950. The marketplace has exploded in growth of demand for housing, cars, clothing, food, utilities, education, entertainment, etc. Another issue is: Are the prices of food, gasoline and housing going up or are you getting more for your dollars? In health care if you can ask are the prices going up, are you asking if we are spending more on individuals or are individuals using more health care? Finally, are we getting more for our dollars?

Many will argue that we spend more because we get more.

In 1950 President Eisenhower was treated for a heart attack with bed rest, first in the hospital for 6 weeks and then at home for 6 months. Six weeks of bed rest at the hospital would cost a fortune today and now there are other treatments that get the patient up and walking in a very short period of time. Vice-president Cheney is a good example. The treatment for depression has also changed. If you have seen the movie "One Flew Over the Cuckoo's Nest" of the 50s you saw how people were warehoused in mental institutions. Today they give those with depression Prozac or Zoloft or some other medication but not hospitalization unless it's for 3 or 4 days to stabilize the suicidal patient. The costs of treatment have gone down. However, today we use medication and psychotherapy, and the number of people being treated has gone up. Therefore, the overall cost of treating depression in the United States has risen due to the greater number of people receiving treatment, not because the hourly rate has risen. It hourly rate of psychotherapy with a master's level professional was $20 in the 1960s. Today Medicaid's reimbursement is $52.51. Twenty dollars in today's marketplace would be at least $100.

We are making a mistake by just looking at the dollars per session. If you want to evaluate the benefits of mental health care you have to ask: Has the value gone up? To answer this question, consider these two benefits: morality and quality of life. While we are living longer, quality of life is much more difficult to measure. If saving a person from a suicidal gesture is saving a life, then what is the yearly value of that person's life if they live another 40 years? What is that worth in the total scheme of health care dollars?

Since we are discussing the value of our health care dollars, consider that the costs of car air bags are $300 to $1500 depending on number of air bags and make of car. The probability of air bags saving your life is about 1 in 10,000 accidents. That may run about $3 to 5 million per life. Per year that may average out to $125,000, depending, of course, the age of the accident victim and if they are prone to accidents. Since there is government support for air bags, then one can assume that $125,000 a year per person it saves from death is worth the cost. (7)

If we are able to help a young First Grader get on medication, then train him or her how to handle their impulsivity and restlessness and concentration problems, is the value calculated with a High School graduation, with graduation from Business or Nursing school, or when the person retires on a adequate pension and doesn't have to rely on Social Security?

If we help a young mother get away from an abusive relationship, is the value of our work calculated with the life of the mother and child? It is the fact that they were able to access appropriate health care? Or maybe the value can be quantified by the fact that there was a therapist who accepted her insurance policy?

How do you calculate the value of psychotherapy and medications for Posttraumatic Stress Disorder? Schizoid Affective Disorder? Panic Attacks? Bi-Polar Disorder? Paranoid Schizophrenia? We have yet to calculate these disorders in economic value to the community. But we must! Because that is how the policy makers think, talk and make decisions about our field of study.

Given the choice between health care and groceries, a majority of people may choose the short-term answer. The government's top advisors and policy writers will ask the same question. And they will get the same answer. The top advisors have worked in

"Think tanks", universities, in a variety of corporate organizations but they are not health care providers. They have experience with HMOs and PPOs, not one minute of experience in a rural community health center as a provider or as a private practice provider. The bottom line overrides any clinical symptom. Politians and employers want more bang for THEIR dollar so they are more likely to look at their bottom line (dollars and voters), not the worth of our services to society.

Health care is a business. If you have your own company, you are an entrepreneur. The first thing practitioners can do is change their point of view. We need to understand, appreciate and discuss the value of our work. For clinicians the dominating priority is the health of the patient. For entrepreneurs the dominating priority is the matter of gain or loss. Creative accounting can sometimes delay an expect loss, but a loss can not be just "written-off as an expense or an experience" as many non entrepreneurs often mistakenly believe. Accounting is a check and balance of the units of goods, services, and money. It speaks not to serviceability or mechanical efficiency of the goods and services. The base line of every organization is the related in terms of money values. The entrepreneur views his/her company in terms of ownership and ownership in terms of money. Investments of capitalization for personnel, equipment, real estate or some other form of expansion is judged by bankers, accountants and entrepreneurs in terms of the value of the dollar unit, and wither it yields a profit or not. All investments (start-ups or expansion) are made with the assumption that the investor (entrepreneur) is going to make a profit, given that the marketplace continues in a stable and orderly increase and the business traffic to his/her company will also increase. For the many, clinicians think first and foremost of the patient and not of the expenses and liabilities of therapy.

A second stumbling block to understanding the value is the matter of waste. From the entrepreneur's perspective there is waste. Therapists and social workers and staff members who think they are working for the government tend to show-up, drink coffee, contribute to the rumor mill, and collect their checks. That may work in large organizations, but not is small companies. Although one would like to believe that all medical and mental health employees are devoted to their professions, it just isn't so. The passion isn't there. Their attitude is aggressive and turf-protective. They may be pleasant with patients but unreliable when it comes to doing all they can to increase the bottom-line. It's not their problem, it's yours. They do not understand the value of therapy or medicine, and they certainly do not understand the value of provider time. Every minute of every day there are costs accumulating: payroll costs, operating costs, fixed costs, variable costs, they all add up and most be accounted for and someone must be responsible for them. When a health care provider settles for less, the value of his/her services decreases and the costs go up, for the company, the patient and for society.

A third obstacle is not having a good support staff. Setting up appointments, calling patients to remind them of appointments, ensuring that each patient has insurance or is paying cash, ensuring that each patient understands the rules of confidentiality are critical limits in a business and helps the providers reach their practice goals. When people do not show up for their appointment, or re-schedule frequently, the business suffers. When in-house billers are underpaid and overworked they can commit errors which might not be caught for two or three months. This will delay revenue which adds costs. If the billing is done in such as way that it attracts an audit, there are legal costs and liabilities. Having an educated, experienced staff adds value to the practice and contributes significantly to the quality of health care.

A final value not often recognized, but certainly debated especially in utilization reviews or quality assurance programs, is the value of performance. We need to perform in order to heal broken lives. And we, as a society needs to value this performance and pay more appropriate reimbursement rates, perhaps giving bonus' or paying higher rates to those who can document greater effects from their services. And we need to find a way that reflects this value and these effects on society. Documentations lead to justification which can have value for policy makers. Even with out these values and performance adding to the quality of health care and reducing future expenditures, policy makers still need to be persuaded to listen and understand what we do, why we do it, and the value it has to society. The problem, however, still remains; the one with the deepest pockets calls the shots.

Health Care as a Right

It is estimated that one in every four people needs our services. Forty or more million Americans are without health insurance at some point during this year. Given the Oklahoma bombings, 9-1-1 terrorists' attacks, the natural disasters such as earthquake, floods, and hurricanes has given us wake-up calls of our human fragilities and the vulnerability we, Americans, face in the world. We, as a nation, and as health care providers are ill prepared for such disasters. And it doesn't help when our government agencies are attempting to shut us down or reduce our billings to a point where we lose money just by opening the front door of our offices.

To meet the mental health challenge, our political leaders need to create the federal disaster funding to local communities BEFORE a disaster to ensure training and availability. According to Michael M. Faenza, CEO, National Mental Health Association, the coordinated prevention and training programs should focus on providing services to those at risk and identification and treatment of mental health problems. "The American economy is already losing an estimated $113 billion a year from untreated and mistreated mental illness. We cannot afford to let the lingering discrimination and stigma against mental illness stand in the way of meeting this serious public health crisis." (8)

In some states it may be a crime not to render aid at the scene of a car accident. But what about some one that crumbles to the ground coughing, clutching their arm or chest? Do we have the legal or moral obligation to render assistance? Most people in America would certainly jump in, irregardless if there is a Good Samaritan Law or not. There are plenty of stories of people reaching out and helping without asking for anything in return. I've been helped while stranded in the middle of no where, and I've tried to help others in like situations. But if you own stock in a pharmaceutical company that sells medication to people at a price that most can not afford, are they denying people the assistance they need to live or at least that would decrease pain and suffering? Would a pharmacist, be in violation of any legal or moral code for refusing a snakebiten victim the antidote that was needed to survive even if the victim had no money?

Offering health care to everyone is not just a question of spending more money. "At present, the U.S. spends some $2 trillion a year on healthcare, said Michael Dukakis, the former governor of Massachusetts and an advocate for healthcare reform. This expenditure surpasses that of all other countries." (9) The U.S. is ranked 21st in the world in terms of overall healthcare quality. According to the article, the uninsured pays 35% of their healthcare costs and that every family pays about $1200 a year for health care services for the uninsured patient. Mr. Dukakis also argued that policy could not be divorced from politics.

Lessons From Katrina

The catastrophic disaster and images of Hurricane Katrina in August 2005 will forever be sketched deep into the minds of millions of people in the United States. Long before the last person was evacuated fingers were being pointed to various people in authority blaming them for various personal and community losses. One of the objects of attention has been the levee that was built to withstand a Category 3 Hurricane. When Hurricane Katrina hit New Orleans she was a Cat (Category) 5. It didn't take long for the levee to break and all of New Orleans, which sits several fee below sea level, become flooded, up to 9 feet in some places, especially buildings (homes, offices, stores, casinos). Thousands were trapped. Most of these people either couldn't or wouldn't leave New Orleans. It wasn't long before bodies were found floating in streets, their homes, or in ditches. There are many lessons can be learned from disasters like Katrina, that can apply to the chaos surrounding the health care system.

Lesson One: It was predicted four years before it occurred. "In early 2001 experts from the Federal Emergency Management Agency set out to rank the likeliest, most catastrophic disasters facing America. According to the Houston Chronicle, they were a terrorist attack in New York, a major earthquake in San Francisco, and a major hurricane in New Orleans." (10) The Corps of Engineers New Orleans District has spent about $250 million over the past 4 years but it was not enough. Now it will cost billions to bring back New Orleans. Being prepared requires plans and money and tenacious leaders. And yet things can happen that either was not expected or happened at a time when people were not prepared, or by having weak leadership

Lesson Two: The attitude that the big storm or event will happen to someone else, not to you. This storm was a tropical storm and barely a Category 2 when it went over Florida and slowed down over before hitting the very warm waters of the Gulf of Mexico. The way it developed, the slow speed, and the suggestion it would go up the western coast of Florida allowed people to take a less than serious attention to it. Even the day before it hit, there was time to get out but people still stayed. Maybe they thought that their house wouldn't get destroyed or didn't believe the whole city would get such high water. For health care providers, we often take for granted that our services are invaluable and that patients and policy makers would understand that.

Lesson Three: When a crisis occurs health care providers are among the first to be called to help. But between crisis health care providers often are neglected and made to feel that they are the cause of rising health care. During a recent crisis in San Antonio, Texas, the child protective agency was losing people and having employees not do their job. As a result, children were dying, killed by their care givers, which were often a relative or a boyfriend of a parent. Governor Perry rushed in with the promise of hiring needed staff and brining in a group to help define the problems and needs. In a fairly short time a lot of people were hired. They were not licensed professionals, most had only a bachelor level degree often in criminal justice, education, history, political science, etc. None understood or appreciated the need to collaborate with community professionals. They have stepped on the toes of many professionals, ordering and badgering and bulling their way through their daily tasks. At times they have been known to mislead or deliberately mislead professionals, and in some cases when the professionals did not agree with them, the unlicensed case worker has written letters of complaint to the licensed professional's board. This has created a great deal of mistrust and antagonism in the health care community. These attitudes are compounding the effect of the present crisis in health care.

A survey taken of New Yorkers on their attitudes and fears since 9-1-1 found that "fears over terrorism remain prevalent among New York City residents. Fifty-two percent think about the possibility of a future attack occurring in the city. Fifty-eight percent worry that they or someone they know will become the victim of terrorism. Women (66 percent vs. 47 percent of men) are more likely to be worried about victimization from terrorism. Thirty-one percent of citizens feel less safe than they did after the 9/11 terrorist attacks, while 47 percent feel as safe as they did after the attacks. Now nearly four years later, only 21 percent feel safer.

"Safety of various modes of transportation is of serious concern. Subway riders feel the least safe. Fifty-two percent of subway riders and 51 percent of train riders do not feel safe while commuting in New York City. The recent London bombings promoted flashbacks of 9/11 among New York City residents. Forty-eight percent experienced a flashback including 52 percent of women and 44 percent of men. Eighty-five percent think that groups similar to the London bombers exist in New York City today." (11)

ೞ೮ಲ

Power Point

With the advent of managed care has come the emphasis on justification of the need for care, cost effectiveness and efficiency, and the increasing need to create a defensive strategizing posture in the administration and delivery of health care. Therefore, where else might such education start except in graduate school? However, the real test of character and compassion will come soon after the graduate becomes a health care provider. Shattered expectations can be replaced with a growing sense of inner balance and hope as you gain experience from being flexible, creative and innovative and committed to compassionate quality health care.

End of Chapter Review

Multiple Choice Questions

1. Society has not kept up with the growth and development of psychotherapy services, such as issues of:
   a. Ethics
   b. Environment
   c. Financing
   d. Infrastructure
   e. A, C, D

2. The Colonial Hills Hospital Case Study alleged that the hospital was crediting a scheme to make fraud by paying an outside company to transport patients to the hospital without a doctor seeing them first, and
   a. Billing too much for their services
   b. Not getting pre-authorizations first
   c. Not hiring licensed medical doctors
   d. Letting the insurance coverage determine what services the patient received and for how long they stayed rather than the medical necessity.

3. Health care providers of all disciplines can use this book to build a framework of understanding of the business side of health care and the:
   a. Issues an entrepreneur encounters
   b. Problems patients face every day in doctor offices
   c. Challenges of dealing with incurable diseases or disorders
   d. Limitations of graduate school curriculums

4. The rational for this book includes:
   a. The costs of practicing therapy and health care are increasing.
   b. With managed care and recent state budget priority changes, there is a decrease in populations that can receive our services.
   c. The costs of practicing therapy and health care are increasing

        d. There is a lack of information about the business side of therapy

        e. All the above

5. At the core of our basic presentation to our patients are:
        a. The costs of liability and risks
        b. Our values and beliefs
        c. Medical necessities
        d. If they have insurance or not

Rethink

1. What have you studied in either undergraduate or graduate school about the business side of health care?
2. What are the key points of this chapter?
3. How will this book help you prepare for the practice of medicine or therapy?
4. After reading this chapter how has your expectations of practice changed?

Personal Observations

1. Discuss with a licensed health care provider (who has been in practice more than five years) how they survived their fist few years of practice.
2. Discuss with a practicing therapist or medical health care provider about how they handle the business side of health care.
3. Research how bureaucrats and entrepreneurs different in practice of their discipline.

Chapter References

1. Hixson, Ronald R., The Business of Therapy: The Need to Educate Therapists in the Business Aspects of Practice, Annals, Journal of the American Psychotherapy, Summer 2004, Volume

7, Number 2.

2. Broskowski, Anthony, Current Mental Health Care Environments: Why Managed Care Is Necessary, p. 13, The Mental Health Professionals Guide to Managed Care, Rodney L. Lwman and Robert J. Resnick, Editors, American Psychological Associaiton, Washington, D.C., 1994.

3. Libby, Ronald T., Ph.D., www.healthleaders.com, Oct. 26, 2001

4. Nowlin, Sanford, Swarming Capitol paid off for SBC, San Antonio (TX) Express-News, April 11, 2006, A1 and A8. also read: Gary Scharrer, Lobbying didn't let up when the CHIP was down, San Antonio Express-News, August 14, 2006, A1 and A10.

5. Faenza, Michael M. www.mha-mi.org, 7/6/04

6. Ibid.

7. Cutler, David M., Your Money Or Your Life, Oxford University Press, NY, 2004, p.15. The estimates are from the work of John D. Graham, et al, The Cost-Effectiveness of Air Bags by Seating Position, Journal of the American Medical Association 278, no. 17, (November 5, 1997): 1418-25.

8. Faenza, Michael M. www.mha-mi.org, 7/6/04.

9. Hefler, Janel, Health Care Forum addresses insurance and reform issues, The Martha's Vineyard Times, Martha Vineyard, MA, August 21, 2005, p.1

10. The St. Louis Post Dispatch as quoted in the Caller-Times, Scripps Texas, L.P., Corpus Christi, TX, September 5, 2005, p. 11A

11. Myers, Mike, www.healthpolitics.com, October 9, 2005

Chapter Two
Legal Twisters and Hurricanes

Summary

With the advent of managed care have come increased laws and regulations that affect the nature and spirit of the practice of health care. The whole purpose is to control revenues and services by increasing restrictions on practices. Laws can be used to knock providers out of the business, increasing prosecution tools, limiting access to health care and cutting reimbursements for different procedures to discourage providers from delivering services, thereby reducing health care costs. This chapter will cover the impact of a select few health care laws on the practice of health care.

What you will learn in this chapter:

1. You will be able to expand your awareness of a number of issues that support library full of legislation.
2. You will be provided with a brief introduction to several laws that if ignored, could land you in jail or at the very least cause fines in excess of your salary for three years or longer.
3. You will be introduced to several issues that normally do not affect a solo practitioner but that could affect a joint venture, collaboration, or working relationship.
4. A Case Study will present how you can lose your business/ practice without committing a crime.

Business Law

The practice of law has exploded over the past 25 years. "In 1970, there were about 350 lawyers. By the mid-1980s, there were 650,000". (1) By the 1990s the number of practicing attorneys was estimated over 1 million. Two-thirds of them practiced in America. The number admitted to practice in the 1970s were more than all those admitted to the bar the previous 100 years. "The increase in litigation and in the number of lawyers is consistent with another tend in our society – increased regulation of business. The basic role of law in business decisions is readily apparent. It constrains business in its decisions and in its selection of alternative course of action. Certain conduct is illegal, and individuals or businesses who commit acts or omissions declared to be illegal are subject to sanctions. There may be fines or imprisonment if the conduct is declared a crime. Business decisions must be made within the law, or sanctions will be imposed. The law is the foundation for the regulations of all business conduct and decisions." (2)

Laws are commands by society: You will not kill. You will not break a contract. You will not speed, abuse your children or set your house on fire. Laws command what is considered "good" and proper by society today while defining what is considered "bad" or improper. Courts require compliance by providing a remedy against the party breaking the law. Civil courts do no require compliance, with a few exceptions, and instead impose liability for noncompliance.

"Law is a scheme for controlling the conduct of people; it deals with social interests. Whereby social interests recognize a right in one person, courts create machinery to assist the person with this right in obtaining redress against the person with the duty or obligation, if the duty is not performed or if the obligations are unfulfilled." (3) According to Corley and Reed there are four characteristics to law:

a. A way to control society.

b. It attempts to protect the interests of society.

c. Recognizes the power of people to influence or control the actions or conduct of others.

d. It brings in a place for disagreements are settled in a civil and legal manner: the courts.

Businesses need control for a number of reasons to include reduction of uncertainty, in order to manage materials, resources and employees. To better understand organizational control you can consider congruent values, socialization of participants, and performance appraisals. Another way is to consider the flow of resources, revenues, talented and educated employees, and quality of products made or services performed. "If all key organizational decision makers 'think alike,' the managerial system is very likely 'in control.' The extreme, of course, is some form of brainwashing, wherein individuals come to think in only one extremely narrow way about pertinent issues. Certainly there are cases in which conformity is carried too far. We continue to advocate and respect individual initiative. On the other hand, organizations require group effort; the term itself implies cooperation and compromise on the part of the group members as they attempt to achieve some common purpose." (4)

Behavioral control is only one type of control that organizations employ to improve the bottom line. After all, businesses are created to make money, not lose it. Foundations are created to give money away to certain projects or non-profit organizations. Budgets are a way for an organization to control the effects of everyday stress on companies and the storms of change and the unexpected. Budgetary control is a way to restrict and apply constraint on decisions and actions of the company. Budgets are normally expressed in financial records by accountants and are a way to put realism into planning. Comparative studies of the budget with financial statements are a way to evaluate operational goals and success. Budgets are used as a benchmark for projects and departments. Sales use total sales per month as a way to judge the effectiveness of their sales team, and perhaps of their marketing team, too. Management then uses past quarterly budget to project future growth or stagnation. If a company has several departments and several levels, the department administrators are often asked to be part of the budget process. They do this by determining what their department's needs are for the next fiscal year and adjusting for change or/and market adjustments. Management takes each budget and pencils them to the larger picture, the organization's budget. Each department is allocated a total dollar amount for operating and payroll expenses.

The control factor for businesses is the function of maintaining a focus of activity towards the stated organizational goal and mission. Control is as much a part of the managerial process as planning and organizing. According to Kast and Rosenzweig there are four fundamental elements of a control system:

a. A measurable characteristic
b. A sensor
c. A comparator
d. An effector (5)

Since the law is a way to control society, organizations use the law to control behavior in their "society". Applying these four elements to the law of business one can conclude the following as part of that analogy:

a. A measurement of the effect of a law on an organization is whether or not the organization demonstrates compliance.

b. A sensor of the effect of the law on an organization is someone or something that receives a message or some information of the crossing of the line, such as an allegation of inappropriate harassment, or statement of how a procedure of the organization is may be in violation of a state or federal regulation.

c. A comparator is how a policy, procedure, process, or department or organizational goal compares with that of a competitor.

d. An effector is a way to judge effectiveness. Every organization has some type of quality control or quality assurance.

cs80

Case Study

Not too many years ago a mental health group had about 15 therapists and six staff members. They were billing about 600,000 per year and receiving over 60 referrals a week. Each therapist was averaging 30 billable hours a week. Every Friday they had a general meeting to discuss administrative problems and successes. After an administrative meeting there was a clinical meeting to discuss clinical issues, questions, and issues. At least once a month they held a compliance committee meeting where they would discuss areas of compliance and questions of non-compliance or questionable practices or procedures.

One day they started receiving calls from patients who stated that they had received a letter from the Attorney General questioning the billing dates and times of one of their family members. Each date of billing included how much was billed and how much was paid. The patients wanted to know how to respond and what it all meant. At the next meeting the group discussed it. It was decided to run an inner random audit of cases. Later they started getting calls reporting that their patients were receiving visits by the Attorney General's Office and the FBI. They reported that these agents were claiming that they were going to prosecute for insurance fraud, laundering money, embezzlement and some other charges they didn't understand and that their therapist was going to jail.

At some point received a call from an Investigator from the Attorney General's Office who wanted to talk about some cases. At this point the corporate attorney was called and she called the U.S. Attorney General who handles the prosecution of any state insurance fraud involving federal funds. She was told that the group's owner was "the target" but that he didn't know much about the case at that point. A "target" is the one "going down" per insider informant language.

The owner called me after her attorney said she needed a criminal attorney. She went to one attorney who specialized in health care law and was told that their fee would be $50,000. Since she didn't $50,000 she called another defense attorney who lacked the health care experience the first group had but she could afford his fee. So he called the FBI and they set up a meeting.

At the meeting they assured my attorney that they were not there to arrest the therapist, wanting to discuss some basic questions first, reserving the possibility for an arrest at a later date. Those present included investigator from the Attorney General's office and two FBI agents. They asked questions like, was I surprised to see them, how many people worked for me (I had a list with dates of employment to give to them), some questions about billing, what sources referred to us, and would I be surprise to know that someone was billed over 20 times who reported never seeing me. I denied having billed for anyone I never had seen but couldn't explain how that happened, if it did happen.

The meeting with two about 90 minutes and at the end they asked for copies of all files from a certain date to a recent date (about 5 years of practice), copies of each year's Medicaid books, copies of appointment books, copies of financial statements from the corporation and for my personal financial records, copies of bank statements, compliance committee notes, and weekly billing statements to Medicaid and others. They advised us not to change anything in any progress note or chart or and piece of information for which they asked. A date was made to pick up all the information they requested which was about 10 days from that point. He told me that they could be looking for anything, that his experience was that they would collect the information and go through everything and not to expect to hear from them for several months.

Ten days later they brought a U-Haul truck and packed in about 80 boxes of files and information. Those staff and the few therapists that helped prepare for this date were exceptional supporters and human beings. Eighteen excruciating months dragged by and they heard nothing. Finally, the owner called the FBI and asked if they needed anything else. In a few days the agent called and asked if they could pick up the files.

Now, given this scenario, what would you do differently and why, and what would you do next?

CRSO

Insurance Fraud

Insurance fraud refers to fraud against the insurance industry (including Medicaid and Medicare) and fraud by the insurance industry (those who sell or administrate insurance policies or programs and those who are providers). Fraudulent billing by health care providers also includes unlicensed providers and fraud rings involving health insurance claimants, providers and attorney. Staged burglaries are also a part of insurance fraud. These range from the entire burglary being staged to simple inflations of a claim for a legitimate burglary.

Fraudulent activities can include misuse of funds by officers, directors or other employees of an organization, misuse of funds by a third party administrator, surplus lines insurers and the misuse of customer premiums paid to an insurance agent or attorney. The investigators also conduct allegations of submission of false information on licensing applications and financial statements to the Department of Insurance. Material misstatements on a required filing with the Department of Insurance are a third degree felony in Texas.

According to the Coalition against Insurance Fraud, insurance fraud costs Americans $80 billion each year, and broken down to each family that nearly $1,000 per year. Insurance fraud occurs when people deceive insurance companies, agents or customers/clients/patients by faking an accident, injury, or billing for services not delivered. Fines and penalties for theft and fraud can cost you $25,000 to $250,000 and even more. You can lose your home, your car, your freedom, and your career. The U.S. General Accounting Office estimates that health care fraud costs consumers approximately $35 to $60 billion dollars annually of which health care fraud is only a fraction of the fraud pie. Millions are made off of storms, fake car accidents, and people lying about their present pain levels or their previous injuries on forms or to the doctor and adjustor, patients malingering from injuries sustained at work. These result in higher premiums and out-of-pocket costs for employees and tax payers. (6)

The following are a few examples of actual insurance fraud cases:
1. Knowingly receiving stolen goods and a "chop shop" scheme.
2. Insurance fraud, a 3rd Degree Felony.
3. Insurance Fraud, a State Jail Felony.
4. Misapplication of Fiduciary Property and for Theft, both 1st degree Felonies; and for Forgery, a State Jail Felony.
5. Mail Fraud, aiding and abetting; Money Laundering, aiding and abetting, and conspiracy to defraud.

The following are a few examples of actual case dispositions as reported on the Internet:

1. One year confinement and ordered to pay $3649 in restitution.
2. Thirty-Six months deferred adjudication and 240 hours of community service and ordered to pay $109,423.
3. Thirty-Seven months confinement fined $100 and order to pay $744.672 in restitution.
4. Forty months confinement fined $100 and ordered to pay $1,438,501 in restitution.
5. Thirty months confinement, fined $100, and ordered to pay $230,966.
6. One Hundred and thirty five months confinement, fined $3000, ordered to pay $5,175,774 for one count of Conspiracy to Commit Money Laundering, seven counts of Mail Fraud, seventeen counts of Money Laundering.

In one case a Chicago medical doctor being charged with $15,000,000 restitution for Medicaid fraud. The judge listened to the case and determined that the doctor may be a good doctor but a lousy detail person with his paperwork. He was charged $1200 for court costs.

Three psychiatrists were charged with Medicaid and Medicare fraud involving two Texas mental health centers that served moderate to severe mental retardation and serious mental disorders like schizophrenia. Many of the patients couldn't communicate and sat staring. The doctors were allegedly told to pay up $32 millions and they could continue practicing. They said they didn't have it so they lost their Medicaid and Medicare privileges. One joined the Air Force as a psychiatrist, one was said to have gone to Mexico and the last one has not been seen for several years. A medical case management firm was told that they had to get a $100,000 bond if they wanted to continue operating. If not, they would not be allowed to see patients. Another large organization was allegedly told to pay $50,000 and they U. S. Attorney would drop the case. Each case is different, and all the facts are often eluding us, but the bottom line remains that state and federal officers of the court have enormous power over our futures and our careers with little chance of being supervised by an outside agency or organization.

Health care providers are not the only ones liable for charges of insurance fraud. The large pharmaceutical company, Pfizer, has been accused by a Teamsters union of defrauding the union health insurance fund by orchestrating a campaign to get physicians to prescribe the drug Lipitor for patients with low to moderate heart-disease risk, despite the Federal Drug Administration's recommendation for the use of Lipitor for only high-risk patients due to certain side effects. According to the Wall Street Journal the lawsuit "spotlights the practice of off-label marketing of drugs for uses beyond those approved by regulators." (7)

Health Information (HIPPA) Regulations

This is a fairly new animal on the block. Hospitals have received a lot of attention and a majority of guidelines are met for hospitals. However, private practices are not left out. No matter if you have a one-person office you are still required to change some of your ways of handling, protecting, and storing medical information. Mental health files are part of the medical information that is regulated by HIPPA.

Since the HIPPA regulations were signed into law confidentiality has become a greater liability then it was prior-HIPPA. The range of confidentiality extends from the sign-in of the patient to signing of the forms of consent for care, consent to bill the patient's insurance company, consent to share information with stated parties (school teacher, with their primary care physician, psychiatrist and the psychologist who performed psychological assessment on the child or parent). Some therapist have the patient or parent sign a statement that they are aware that psychotherapy may cause some discomfort, perhaps help them recall some unpleasant memories.

Waivers of confidentiality should be updated periodically, and when a new source is attached or is to be included on the consent to share information form, i.e. with an attorney or child protective services. If you have a question, ask your attorney. HIPPA is such a large Act that it's impossible to do justice to every issue in the Act. For more information about HIPPA attend a continuing education course on line or seminar based, gathers information from your corporate attorney, asks other professionals in the field, or goes to the Internet and choose one of a number of Websites. (8)

When picking out an attorney choose one with a background of health care law, another one for contract specialty, another one for setting-up and registering a trade mark, a corporate expert, and a criminal lawyer who can defend you allegations of fraud. Each aspect is a specialty that can means "life and death" to your practice or group practice. Knowing the difference and seeking out a specialty lawyer for these needs can save you thousands of dollars.

For the typical small practice of health care, the Privacy Rule requires the provider to:

1. Notify patients about their privacy rights and how their information can be used.
2. Adopt and implement privacy procedures for his or her practice.
3. Train employees so that they understand the privacy procedures.
4. Designate an individual to be responsible for seeing that the privacy procedures are adopted and follower.
5. Secure patient records containing individually identifiable

health information so that they are not readily available to those who do not need them.

6.   The scalability of the Privacy Rule allows that the privacy official at a small health care practice can be the office manager who is likely to have many other tasks that are non-privacy related.

7.   The training requirement for small health care practices may be a privacy policy document that all staff members have read and signed. (9)

One of the many questions that private practitioners ask has to do with sign-in sheets. Their concerns have to relate to calling out patients by name and that others will not only see their name on sign-in forms but hear their name called. According to the Privacy Rule policy this is acceptable as long as no health care information about the patient is disclosed.

Another frequently asked question has to do with calling patients at their home and leaving messages with family members or even a "message" phone or on an answering machine. According to the HIPPA Privacy Rule this is also acceptable as long as long as no information about the patient's health is discussed or left with anyone besides the patient. If a patient requests that letters or reminders of appointment be sent in a closed envelope rather than by postcard every effort must be made to accommodate them.

According to the HIPPA Privacy Rule the following types of insurances are not covered under the HIPPA regulation: long/short term disability, workers' compensation, automobile liability that covers medical payments, credit-only insurance coverage for on-site medical clinics, and any other benefits for medical care that are secondary or incidental to other insurance benefits.

The Privacy Rule permits health care providers to disclose protected health care information to another health care provider for treatment purposes. This can be done by fax or by other means. Covered entities must have in place reasonable and appropriate administrative, technical, and physical safeguards to protect the privacy of protected health information that is disclosed using a fax machine. Examples of measures that could be reasonable and appropriate in such a situation include the sender confirming that the fax number to be used is in fact the correct one for the other health care provider's office, and placing the fax machine in a secure location to prevent unauthorized access to the information.

Parents have a right to see their child's medical records if the parent is the personal representative of their child. For example, a child that has been taken away from the home by a state agency may have the agency as their personal representative. Each state may have a different slant of this law. But, generally, there are three situations when the parent would not be the minor's personal representative under the Privacy Rule. These exceptions are:

(1) when the minor is the one who consents to care and the consent of the parent is not required under the state or other applicable law;

(2) when the minor obtains care at the direction of a court or a person appointed by the court; and

(3) when and to the extent that, the parent agrees that the minor and the health care provider may have a confidential relationship. However, the Privacy Rule continues, even in these exceptional situations, the parent may have access to the medical records of the minor related to this treatment when the state or other applicable law requires or permits such parental access. Parental access would be denied when state or other law

prohibits such access. If state or other applicable law is silent on a parent's right of access in these cases, the licensed health care provider may exercise his or her professional judgment to the extent allowed by law to grant or deny parental access to the minor's medical information. (10)

After reading the above, it should become very clear to you that were not alone in the therapy room with the patient anymore. We have several government agencies in the room, if not physically, certainly in spirit and in law. Therefore, it is critical for us to have legal representation from a firm that has more than one health care attorney and who can provider both legal advice for practice, including the formation of appropriate forms, but also one that can defend us against allegations of fraud or unprofessional care or in some way in violation of the Privacy Rule or another rule of which may not be acquainted.

OSHA

Occupational Safety & Health Administration (OSHA) was created to protect workers from unsafe working conditions "by setting and enforcing standards; providing training, outreach, and education; establishing partnerships; and encouraging continual improvement in workplace safety and health". (11) Normally mental health employees' work in an office building without much concern with safety unless it is from patients who may get violent quickly or from a needle that accidentally jabs an employee. However, there are times when patient's family members may get up-set with what is being said and accomplished in therapy.

Stark Amendments

The Stark amendments to the Social Security Act were written to prohibit physicians from referring Medicaid and Medicare patients to health care providers and programs where they have a financial interest.

Congress initiated an imposition of civil penalties for violations of this law. In addition, there are issues of insurance fraud with federal penalties and fines for paying for referrals or receiving any form of "kickback" in exchange for sending referrals to organizations in which they have a financial interest. "The first Stark amendments, passed as part of the Omnibus Budget Reconciliation Act (OBRA) of 1989, prohibited physicians from referring Medicare patients to clinical laboratories when the physician had a financial interest in the lab. The 1989 statute and subsequent modifications provide for several exceptions to the prohibition on referrals based on variation in the ownership/investment and/or compensation arrangements between the physician and the entity providing the designated health services (DHS)." (12) The Stark amendments do not apply to non-federal programs.

Sarbanes-Oxley Act

The "SOX" as it is often referred to as, was introduced at least in part due to the Enron financial and legal problems as well as other large corporation who have investors. This Act introduced stringent new rules with the stated objectives such as "to protect investors by improving the accuracy and reliability of corporate disclosures made pursuant to the securities laws". (13) This Act was created to provide governmental regulations on the accounting industry because of the different creative systems found upon investigation. These were created to confuse and deliberately mislead the financial institutions and investors who depend on them in order to make judgments for offering loans and to recommend investments. The Chief Financial Officer (CFO) generally works with the accounting department to create the financials in order to enhance the corporation's position in the marketplace. President George W. Bush is quoted as claiming that this Act is intended "to deter and punish corruption, ensure justice for wrongdoers, and protect the interests of workers and shareholders." (14) As with most federal laws and regulations, there is a price to pay. First, for large corporations, such as chemical giant W. R. Grace & Co., Inc., the cost to comply can run over a million dollars. Secondly, the Act requires public disclosure of fraud, which "can affect lawyer-client confidentiality. But the American Bar Association moved closer to smoothing over that controversy with its own plan to loosen confidentiality rules. Through corporate fraud will invariably persist, the act will ensure that the public companies that survive increased scrutiny will become stronger, more honest and more worthy of investor capital." (15)

An example of a company managing its own compliance of this Act is KPMG which reported to Australian authorities of an internal investigating of a possible multimillion-dollar fraud allegedly committed by a former partner. The firm suggested that the sum of the fraud was in excess of $2 million. KPMG also reported contacting those clients of their previous partner (who resigned) in order to stem the reputation damaged to the organization. (16)

Workers' Compensation

Workers' Compensation Commission attempts to eliminate fraud within the Workers' Compensation program. The Commission reports that they estimate that millions of dollars are paid out illegally each year. Employers, employees, insurance carriers, and consumers pay the cost of fraud in lost jobs and profit, lower wages and benefits, and higher costs for products, services and insurance premiums. Like their counter parts in the Department of Insurance the Workers' Compensation Commission works with special investigation units to deter fraud assisting the prosecution of those who commit fraud. According to these commissions publicly stated policies, including their purpose and mission, they join with teams of trained agents of state and federal law enforcement, other regulatory agencies, and insurance carrier special investigation units. Investigations by these groups often lead to indictment and often prosecution and recovery of money that has been gained through fraudulent schemes that are committed by employers, employees, health care providers, attorneys, insurance agents and others.

The Texas Workers' Compensation Commission describes "fraud" as occurring "when a person knowingly or intentionally conceals, misrepresents, and makes a false statement to either deny or obtain workers' compensation benefits or insurance coverage, or otherwise profit from the deceit. The key to conviction is proving in court that the misrepresentation or concealment occurred knowingly or intentionally." (17)

Employee fraud indicators include:
- injuries that have no witness other than the worker
- injuries occurring late Friday or early Monday
- injuries not reported until a Week or more after they occur
- worker observed in activities inconsistent with the reported injury
- conflicting diagnosis from subsequent treating doctors

Attorney/health care provider fraud indicators include:
- "boilerplate" medical reports or reports that are merely copies of previously submitted reports.
- bills from a health care provider or attorney that present an unreasonable amount of hours per day.
- treatment dates on holidays for non-emergency situations
- attorney relationship with a health care provider that appears to be a partnership in handling workers' compensation claims.

Employer fraud indicators include:

- payroll information on the insurance application inconsistent with payroll reported to the Workforce Commission
- much larger premium paid for the previous year's policy
- small payroll reported by a large company or employee leasing company
- frequent addition and cancellation of coverage

Whistleblower Protections

The Occupational Safety and health Act (OSHA) was created to achieve a safer workplace in America. In order to be able to help workers, there had to be those who would be willing to provide insider information. The Whistleblower Program forbids discrimination for "blowing the whistle" on dishonest employers. Discrimination may involve any of the following:

- firing or lying off
- assigning to undesirable shifts
- blacklisting
- demoting
- denying of benefits
- disciplining
- denial of benefits
- failure to hire or rehire
- intimidation
- transferring
- reassigning work
- reducing pay or hours (18)

This protection is for anyone who wants to turn-in illegal activities because all other efforts have failed. In fact, there are ads for whistlebloWerers to turn-in their doctor or pharmaceutical company, hospital or financial institution. One ad claims that:

"You may be entitled to Missions of Reporting Fraud at your workplace. If your employer failed to offer state Medicaid agencies at the best price pharmaceuticals, you may be entitled to a large cash award. Acknowledge of other systematic health care fraud may entitle you to collect... Under Federal law a person who brings fraud to the attention of the government share of the amount returned to the government. In March 2005, Dr. Steven Bander who reported systematic fraud at Gambo Health Care will personally collect $56 million dollars for blowing the whistle at these Kidney Dialysis clinics." (19)

Equal Employment Opportunity (EEO)

The landmark legislation of 1960s was the Civil Rights Act of 1964 which was followed by the Equal Employment Opportunity Act (1972). The Equal Employment Commission (EEOC) was created to direct federal enforcement of the act. Briefly, the EEO prohibits discrimination in hiring, firing, payroll, or other conditions of employment due to race, color, religion, sex, or national origin. Today organizations have training programs geared to teach affirmative action programs. The EEO recognizes at least three types of discrimination: (1) disparate treatment, (2) disparate effect, and (3) present effect of past discrimination. Discrimination constitutes different treatment of people of different ethnic, culture, gender, or religion. Disparate effect occurs when any particular practice has an adverse impact upon one of these groups. In 1978 another group was added: pregnant employees. If any allegation is made the employer must prove that it is job related or change or face civil actions by the government. (20)

Employer Regulatory Laws

The following are current personnel regulations affecting most businesses:

Americans with Disabilities Act (ADA

Civil Rights Act of 1991

Civil Rights Act Title VII

Consolidated Omnibus Budget Reconciliation Act (COBRA)

Employee Polygraph Protection Act (EPPA)

Employee Retirement Income Security Act (ERISA)

Equal Pay Act

Executive Order 11246

Fair Labor Standards Act (FLSA)

Federal Unemployment Tax Act (FUTA)

Health Insurance Portability and Accountability Act (HIPAA)

HR 101: Capsule Summaries of the Major HR Laws

Immigration Reform and Control Act (IRCA)

Occupational Safety and Health Act (OSHA)

Pregnancy Discrimination Act

Rehabilitation Act of 1973

The Age Discrimination in Employee Act (ADEA)

Uniformed Services Employment and Reemployment Rights Act

Vietnam Era Veterans Readjustment Act of 1974 (21)

Duty to Warn, Protect

Most state laws require that medical or mental health professionals, including any school official, report any incident of child abuse or neglect. In addition any person who threatens to kill anyone, or is endanger of hurting themselves or committing suicide needs to be shared with parents or appropriate authorities. We have a duty to warn per state law and professional ethical codes.

Unlike duty to warn, which mandates that the therapist consider third parties threatened by patients, duty to protect involves the therapist's responsibility and the limits legal liability in cases of patients who are dangerous to themselves. Duty to protect is variously known as *duty to prevent or duty to commit.* (22) This duty can get tricky if you are working with a patient who is depressed and angry and is suicidal even though they do not say they are. Therapists act passively and do nothing could be in serious trouble legally if that patient attempts or succeeds with a suicidal gesture. Having a network that includes psychiatrists and a hospital which has a behavioral/psychiatric ward help in getting him/her immediate help like having the patient taken to an emergency room.

Subpoenas

Subpoenas offer a different set of circumstances that challenges therapist-patient relationships. If your patient's attorney sends the subpoena the attorney will normally enclose a release of waver of confidentiality. If another attorney requests a patient's records, call the patient and then consult with her or his attorney. The therapist has an obligation to warm the patient of any embarrassing or incriminating information. Once confidentiality is waived, and you are asked to testify, you will be cross examined. If you are called to testify, you are obligated to tell the truth. If you add to the progress notes, or not reveal what you are asked, you could be held in contempt or accused of perjury.

Before testifying the therapist has an obligation to study the progress notes but also the professional ethics not to white-out or change your notes. It is embarrassing to be asked about the notes and you forget what you wrote or what was covered. When questioned on the witness stand do not embellish or add anything that is not asked. Too frequently therapists add too much which only confuses your statement and could do harm to your patient. Also remember that the courtroom is NOT the place to add your personal speculations. Think about the question, do jump to an answer, and give a thoughtful and honest response. If you don't know, don't remember say so.

If you go through a disposition phase, your statements are subject to be questioned in court. If you wrote a book or journal article(s) about the subject expect to be asked questions about them if relevant about the case. Defense attorneys are expected to disqualify a witness or discredit their statement. Don't take it personally. They are just doing their job.

Privileged Communications

A subpoena does not waive the patient-therapist privilege of communications. Check with your attorney and with your ethical standards for clarification. It is the responsibility of every health care provider to protect the confidentiality of client communications in an ethical and legal manner. Confidentiality called a "privilege" in most legal proceedings. Up to 1828 only attorney-client relationship had this type of privileged communications. In 1828 New York legislators granted this privilege to physician-patient. At some point such privileged communication was adopted for husband-wife, priest/rabbi/minister and parishioners and psychotherapist and patient.

"A subpoena is an order, issued by a court of law, with requires you to appear in person at a certain date and time. Except as described in this recording, you have no legal choice but to appear at the place on the date and time listed on the subpoena. The subpoena may require you to go to court or to an attorney's office to answer questions under oath about a particular case." (24) In most states privilege exists, but it is held by the clients, securing their right to prevent confidential communications from being disclosed in the course of a legal proceedings. In the health care field when a patient invokes privilege, the mental health professional is legally (and ethically) bound to a certain extent, and your attorney will clarify the boundaries. There are exceptions which your attorney will explain. There are a number of situations where privilege does not hold and the health care professional would be well advised to consult with their state law or company attorney.

Professional, Personal and Business Liabilities

Health care work demands personal involvement with patients and often their families. Physical and emotional pain evokes certain fears and anxiety in many patients. They don't like some of these fears and may have a knee-jerk reaction to run or cry. Some blame their physical therapist, chiropractor, medical doctor or psychotherapist. Some have been known to call a complaint into the Examining Board for their doctor or therapist's licensing. There is always the chance that most of us will be held personally responsible for some alleged malpractice, error or mistake. It isn't that we have committed a crime or even used poor judgment in what is suggested to the patient. May be the patient doesn't really want to return to work or take a more active role in their recovery. Maybe they don't want to return to work. Many are afraid their families will make fun of them when they learn that the pain can be reduced with "mind games".

Professional Boards are neither friendly nor cooperative with those they license. Often they make you feel as if you have to prove your innocence and they don't have to really prove your quilt. Several professionals that I know have gone through this process. None have lost their license but all wanted to throw the license back to the Board. In most cases it takes a year to investigate and present the alleged charges to the Board. During that year you may have to renew your license and you'll have to write an explanation for your actions. You can not go wrong by buying professional liability insurance from an organization that has a built-in legal fee reimbursement for just such occasion. Without it you might pay $1,000 or $5,000 up front. Lawyers do not have a payment plan unless you count the "up front" payment option as a plan.

Buying liability insurance a very prudent way to manage risks. Business liability helps cover potential liabilities at the office or in the building leading up to the office to include the elevator. It's not that you might lose a court case, but that your attorney will attempt to settle with the aggrieved party, something most providers cringe at. Business liability can cover your exposure in the parking lot, in the building and in your office. General or premises liability exposure refers to some one slipping on water in the hallway, part of the ceiling falling down on the patient, or the elevator breaks down between floors. If you are the landlord you would purchase general or premises liability insurance. "Third party" coverage pays for claims filed by third parties, not by the insured.

Then there is vicarious liability, which refers to the liability caused by an employee or agent. Loosely based on the legal issue "Responeat Superior", the therapists (or Master) are responsible for the employees, contract providers or patient (Servant). Liability for MCOs and HMOs has been expanded in some courts under the theories of "respondent superior". "This doctrine states that a higher authority is responsible for the actions taken on its behalf. When the providers are direct employees of an HMO (or MCO) it is not difficult to find the HMO (or MCO) liable for employees' misdeeds." (25)

Building liability for any and all furniture, paper, desks, etc., is covered under a fire and theft insurance policy. Your insurance agent will want to know how you have owned this business and how much value do you place on the office contents and furnishings. Take pictures of everything!

Corporate Compliance Programs

Normally legal firms who advertise as health care law as a specialty may not be telling the entire story. You want an agency that has many years of experience conducting corporate compliance audits and the subsequent design and implementation of compliance programs for health care providers, suppliers and insurers of every size and type. Their program methodology should be comprehensive, encompassing compliance standards and procedures, oversight responsibilities, appropriate delegation, employee training, monitoring and auditing, enforcement and discipline, and response and prevention. A well-balanced health care legal team will have experts on the team who can do research compliance; create policies and procedure manuals for institutional review boards, including patient privacy and conflict of interest policies and forms. Some legal agencies have someone who has conducted major internal investigation and prepared a detailed response to allegations of non-compliance issued by the Office for Human Research Protections (OHRP).

Liabilities of Website, Mergers, Acquisitions, Reorganizations and Joint Ventures

Complying with the myriad laws and ethical rules that may apply (such as state and federal privacy regulations or state licensure and corporate practice of medicine rules) can be a very big obstacle. It is hard to compete effectively in today's marketplace without at least considering mergers, acquisitions and reorganizations or joint ventures. To do these legal procedures they have to have expertise in corporate, reimbursement, antitrust, DON and licensure, real estate, pension and employee benefits, tax, fiduciary and other legal issues that arise in such transactions.

A legal team assist clients in establishing a wide variety of joint ventures, including: a joint venture for home health services among a hospital, a visiting nurse association and a durable medical equipment company; a joint venture for ambulance services between a hospital and an ambulance company; joint ventures for multi-hospitals with an imaging services; a joint venture for the construction and sale of condominium units in medical office buildings; various joint venture or partnerships with physician and other health care practitioners, including single and multi-specialty independent practice associations.

ᎷᎾᎾ

Case Study

Look at what a mess the founders and leaders of Enron created. While they made themselves billionaires, they did it on the backs those who were unsuspecting and vulnerable. Some of their leaders may have been sent to prison by the time of this publication, or may find themselves there shortly. Enron was a successful company that may come out of the financial and legal dilemmas as a new but smaller company. The accounting firm that helped with the creative accounting and the misleading financial statements has lost millions and may some of their personnel may end up in prison.

ᎷᎾᎾ

Case Study

Perhaps the most famous hospital Medicaid fraud case, at least in Texas, occurred in 1991 when a 14-year-old boy was taken to Colonial

Hills Psychiatric Hospital in San Antonio. Reports of the case suggested that two hulking uniformed men, who appeared to be police officers, went to the home of the grandparents (legal guardians) to escort the boy to the hospital because of allegations of substance abuse and possible suicidal ideations. The boy was said to be truant from school, had failing grades, was violent and excessively aggressive and was considered by a doctor of being in serious harm to him self. Even though the boy's brother and the grandparents collaborated much of this information, they attempted to gain the boy's release from the hospital after several days. When they were rebuffed by the doctor and the hospital, they went to a U. S. Congressman who was also an attorney, who gained his release. This case led to a multitude of investigations in the psychiatric hospital field. It didn't help that the doctor was not a licensed doctor and had no license to practice medicine. This case was considered a Medicaid fraud case because among other charges, the hospital was alleged to have committed fraud by hiring outside companies to pickup "patients" and take then to the hospital. This was viewed, in part, as paying for referrals. The insurance companies were alleging that the hospital was billing for services when there was no medical necessity, that the length of stay was predicated on how long their insurance would pay and not on the medical necessity.

They Attorney General argued that no doctor admitted the boy was into the hospital, as was required, and that several days went by before the admitting "doctor" interviewed him. Since that time a number of psychiatric hospitals have been closed and mental health and substance abuse inpatient and some outpatient programs shut-down. "On June 29, 1994, National Medical Enterprises, Inc. (NME), agreed to pay a record $379 million in criminal fines, civil damages, and penalties to settle the largest health care fraud case in U.S. history. At one time, NME owned more than 70 psychiatric and substance abuse hospitals in addition to several score of rehabilitation and acute care hospitals." (26) Consequences of this case led to a shortage of inpatient mental health and substance abuse programs and beds. Another consequence has been the stop of payment for legitimate bills for mental health and substance abuse inpatient programs.

CREW

These cases are examples of two businesses, one medical and one non-medical, that have created schemes or/and policies that have led to billions of dollars going into corporate and corporate leadership pockets. This practice, has come back to be their demise. There are thousands of cases of individuals in every state who have attempted to "get over" on someone or some insurance company, or who have created a way to over-bill or to make millions illegally. It is only logical that when entering a field of practice that one does due diligence by gathering as much information about the field or/and the company one is joining or entering. When you invest thousands of dollars and years of study to gain a license, it only makes sense to "buy" insurance (information) that can protect you against various liabilities that can threaten your practice.

CREW

Case Study

More than a few times an unlicensed caseworker doesn't agree with what a licensed therapist has done, so they write letters to the Board of Examiners or help the patient write the complaint letter. A complaint often takes up to 12 months to settle the case. In the mea time the therapist ends up paying higher rates of liability and attorney fees to help them with the Board. In one case that I'm aware of the Board cleared the therapist and then the claimant called a local television hotline and filed a complaint, thus starting a whole new series of embarrassing events.

While providers are attempting to work with their Board, these small bands of "midnight marauders" seldom just close the case. Even when the person has been cleared, they have been known to write a letter of "caution" to the provider. While there may be a number of agencies bending over backward to work with CPS there are medical doctors and social workers and professional counselors refusing to take case from CPS. So now practitioners have to re-learn how to practice therapy, and learn a defense posture. For many, this has been too much, and so they turn to a cash-only practice, or a part-time practice, or go into another field like real estate.

CR8O

Power Point

Liabilities translate into "costs" (financial, ethical, legal, and emotional). Costs destroy budgets, careers, families, practices, and it isn't just the ones who have committed a crime, it hurts innocent partners, employees, family members and everyone that depends on the provider for services. Finally, you don't have even have to be charged with any infraction of the law or professional ethical standards to suffer financial losses or/and the loss of one's reputation.

CR8O

End of Chapter Review

Multiple Choice Questions:

1. According to this chapter the whole purpose of managed health care is to:
    a. Sell more health insurance policies.
    b. Control revenues and services.
    c. Build more affordable hospitals.
    d. Shape health care behavior of the population served.

2. _____ has/have been in the business of creating laws that restrict access to homes and offices, other facilities and to drugs and medications for a long time.
    a. Presidents
    b. Chief Executive Officers (CEOs)
    c. Judges
    d. Government

3. Laws are commands by:
    a. Judges
    b. Government
    c. Legislators
    d. Society

4. Businesses need control for a number of reasons, to include:
    a. Reduction of uncertainty
    b. In order to manage materials
    c. Managing resources and employees
    d. All the above
    e. B and C

5. Unlike duty to warn, which mandates that the therapist consider third parties threatened by patients, duty to protect involves:
    a. The therapist's responsibility and the limits to her or his legal liability in cases of patients who are dangerous to themselves.
    b. A duty to call the police.
    c. A duty to call their parents.

       d. A duty to notify a patient's family and have them commits your patient to a psychiatric ward in an acute care hospital.

6. Waivers of confidentiality should be updated:
   a. Periodically
   b. Monthly
   c. Weekly
   d. Every three years

Rethink

1. When is confidentiality not a privilege?
2. Discuss the role of the Stark Amendments and how it has impacted physicians.
3. Explain how HIPPA enhances communication security for health care patients.
4. Define Medicaid fraud. Can anyone be alleged to have committed Medicaid or insurance fraud?
5. Discuss what a "whistleblower" is and how he or she is protected by the government.

Personal Observation Exercise

1. Go to the internet and pull-up Privacy of Health Information/ HIPPA, specifically the frequently asked questions (FAQ): http//www:ansWerers.hhs.gov. Read the questions and answers. Visit a local health care provider and ask him or her how this legislation has impacted his or her practice.
2. Talk to an attorney who reports experience in health care law. Ask him or her how long he or she has been practicing law, how long he or she has practicing health care law, and what he or she visions to be health care's next great threat to the practitioners' autonomy and financial success.

References

1. Corley, Robert N. and O. Lee Reed, **The Legal Environment of Business**, 7ᵗʰ Ed., McGraw-Hill Book Company, NY, 1987.

2. Ibid, pp. 2 – 3.

3. Ibid, p. 4.

4. Kast, Fremont E. and James E. Rosenzweig, p. 451-452, **Organization And Management**, McGraw-Hill, New York, 1979.

5. Ibid, p. 465.

6. Coalition against Insurance Fraud, www.insurancefraud.org

7. Wilke/Hensley, Wall Street Journal, March 28, 2006, reported in the Kaiser Daily Health Policy Report, Prescription Drugs, March 28, 2006, www.kaisernetwork.org

8. www.simplifiedtraining.com (tools and training); www.manager.com; www.hipaaclickandcomply.com; www.hhs.gov/ocr/hipaa.

9. HIPPA Privacy Rule, www.hhs.gov/ocr/hippa/guidelines/overview.pdf Also at: www.hhs.gov/ocr/privacysummary.rtf and www.cms.hhs.gov/HIPAAGenInfo

10. Ibid.

11. OSHA's Mission, U.S. Department of Labor, www.osha.gov

12. Carrie J. Davidson, Submitted in Partial Fulfillment of Requirements in HSMC 456: Issues in Health Management, Spring 2001

13. Ibid.

14. The Sarbanes-Oxley Act Community Forum, p. 1, www.sarbanes-oxley-forum.com, October 13, 2005; also Sarbanes-Oxley Center: The Act and Strategies for Compliance, PriceWaterhouseCoopers, www.pwcglobal.com

16. Baltimore Business Journal, Baltimore, Maryland, August 18, 2003, p. 1

17. Urban, Rebecca, The Age Company, Ltd., www.theage.com.au/news, March 28, 2006.

18. Texas Workers' Compensation Commission, www.twcc.state.tx.us

19. Whistleblower Regulations, www.whistlebloWerer-qui-tam.com/pages/medicaid.html

20. Ibid.

21. Equal Employment Opportunity Commission, www.eeoc.gov and www.adaportal.org/Other Agencies/EEOC/EEOC TOC.html

22. www.psychlaws.org/LegalResources/statelaws/Delawarestatute.htm

23. Earle, Ralph H., and Dorothy J. Barnes, **Independent Practice for the Mental Health Professional**, Brunner/Mazel Publishers, Philadelphia, 1999, pp. 116-118.

24. What is a Subpena?, www.floridabar.org/tfb/TFBConsum.nsf also Gross, Bruce Privileged Communication, May/June, Annuals 2002, American Psychotherapy Association, p. 1

25. Higuchi, Shirley Ann, Recent Managed-Care Legislative and Legal Issues, p.96, **The Mental Health Profession's Guide to Managed Care**, Rodney L. Lowman and Robert J. Resnick, Editors, American Psychological Association, Washington, D.C., 1994.

26. Kiefer, J. Richard & Carol A. Glass, Defending Charges of Health Care Fraud, The Champion, National Association of Criminal Defense Lawyers, Sept/Oct 1994, p. 1, www.nacdl.org/CHAMPION/ARTICLES

Chapter Three
Ethical Quagmire

Summary

This chapter attempts to increase your awareness of some basic ethical concepts related the practice of health care. To start, this chapter suggests that health care academic programs should look for ways to improve patient-doctor or client-therapist communications and sensitivity. This refers to clinicians being more aware of and sensitive to individuals from different cultural backgrounds, with different primary languages, with different sexual orientations, from different religious backgrounds and with varying religious attitudes, and those with different personal values and beliefs. This chapter also discusses several key areas that relate to religious values, business ethics, and social policies such as the changing biomedical research and its practical and ethical implications. Finally, this chapter offers some ways to deal with unethical behavior, public scandals, including advice on how to develop an ethics program in your practice or organization.

What you will learn in this chapter:

1. You will learn the difference between principlism and casuistry and why this important in the study of ethics.
2. You will come to understand how ethical issues can be challenged by circumstance.
3. You will learn how health care providers can be trained to be more understanding and compassionate, thereby improving the quality of health care they provide.

4. You will be exposed to the business side of managed care and will learn how it affects the clinical side of care in both negative and positive ways.
5. You will also be exposed to several social policies that challenge ethical behavior for health care providers.

The Code

Each license has an ethics requirement, as do most insurance contracts. Ethics requirements are often vague simply because it is difficult to regulate some actions. Most licensing boards specify certain behaviors as being clearly unethical: having sex with a patient, having a dual relationship with a patient or a patient's family, or not reporting a patient's intent to harm him or herself or others. However, a code of ethics cannot specify every action that would be considered unethical. Instead the code provides general guidelines for ethical conduct.

State licensing boards have a duty to "protect the public." Their duty is not to protect those who are licensed under their board's guidelines and authority. They are not an association, club, or professional support system. They are usually made up of people who are not even licensed by that board, though they will have a member or two who are licensed by that board or a different board. All the rules that are incorporated in a state licensing board's code of ethics are there to protect the public against the licensees, and some for very good reasons. For example, despite extremely explicit codes of ethics, licensed professional are still being caught having sex with patients, having dual relationships, etc.

The Texas Administrative Code of Ethics (The Code) is one example of the type of codes of ethics that practitioners will have to conform to. This code admonishes its licensed personnel "not to knowingly make any misleading, deceptive, fraudulent or exaggerated claim or statement about their license, background, training, experience, education, professional affiliations, fees or publications." (1) The code also warns the licensees that they should not make any "exaggerated claim or statement" about the services of a mental health organization; and that the licensees will reframe from making any "exaggerated claim or statement" about the effectiveness of their service.

What many do not know or remember, because it is not talked about in many continuing education courses on ethics, is the responsibility of the licensees to stop others from making false statements or claims, or misrepresenting health care services. The licensees are required to "make reasonable efforts to prevent others whom the licensee does not control from making misrepresentations...and shall take immediate and reasonable action to correct the statement." (2)

This code also states that you, as a therapist, must do the following during the first session with each new patient (or the patient's parents): A licensee shall inform in writing the following:

- fees and arrangements for payment
- therapy purposes, goals, techniques
- any restrictions placed on the license
- the limits of confidentiality
- any intention of using another individual to provide treatment intervention to the patient or family
- and any supervision of the therapist by another licensed therapist, including the qualifications of that supervising therapist (3)

As an additional step, after you put all of this information in writing, it is a good idea to sign and date it, having the responsible party(s) sign(s) it as well. Additionally, the code requires the licensee to provide health care in a professional manner. However, it is hard to have a professional attitude when the patient abuses the provider's time by coming in late or not calling to reschedule until later in the day (if he or she calls at all). While we can not charge Medicare or Medicaid for a no-show charge or a reschedule charge (for either not showing up for the appointment or calling within 24 hours of the scheduled appointment, both of which costs appointment "holes") most third party payers allow for this charge (normally $25) and you have several options:

1. Double book the patient next time (this can be done by scheduling 2 patients at one time slot or scheduling them halfway between two appointments.

2. Call the case manager and explain how your patient is missing x number of times. Some case managers will call the patient and encourage them to not miss any more appointments. Another issue here, especially for Medicaid or Medicare patients is that if the patient continues missing appointments they may lose their insurance coverage for their stated health issue or disorder.

3. Fire yourself (give them three names of other providers)

4. Tell them that there are no openings until next month and if they miss that one, you will not reschedule any others for them.

The next general ethical issue for providers is making any falsification of licensing materials or diagnosing a patient without seeing him or her. In addition, there are the issues of over treating (treating the patient indefinitely, even after the goals of therapy have been met. "A licensee may not persistently or flagrantly over-treat a client." (4)

The Texas Administrative Code has separate sections on proper conduct and misconduct regarding sexual activities with a patient, testing of a patient, the use of drugs and alcohol, confidentiality, licensees and the Board (a licensee must cooperate with the Board, not interfere with investigations, and not file a complaint in bad faith); assumed names, consumer information, advertising and announcements, research and publication, finding of non-fitness for licensure subsequent to issuance of license (such as having a drug or alcohol problem), and finally a section requiring the reporting of child abuse or neglect; the abuse, neglect or exploitation of elderly; and any "abuse, neglect, illegal, unprofessional or unethical conduct in an inpatient mental health facility, a chemical dependency treatment facility, or a hospital providing comprehensive medical rehabilitation services." (5)

Health care providers have a responsibility to their patients. While each licensed and discipline has their own code of ethics, most include the following:

- Providing service without discrimination on the basis of race, age, ethnicity, socioeconomic status, disability, gender, health status, religion, national origin, or sexual orientation;
- Obtaining appropriate informed consent prior to therapy;
- Avoiding any position that would exploit the therapist's position in the therapeutic relationship, i.e., dual relationships;
- Avoidance of any sexual intimacy;
- Compliance with all applicable laws regarding the reporting of any alleged unethical conduct;
- Respecting the rights of patients to make their own decisions;
- Obtaining written informed consent from patients before videotaping, audio recording, or permitting third-party observations;
- Making the nature of the relationship and the limits of confidentiality clear at the start of the relationship;
- Maintaining adequate knowledge of and adhering to applicable laws, ethics, and professional standards;
- Transferring, storing, or disposing of confidential information and records in ways that maintain confidentiality and safeguard

the integrity of the practice and welfare of the patient;

- Not accepting kickbacks, or other remuneration for referrals. (6)

An ethical issue that is <u>not</u> addressed by the ethical standards of licensing boards is when a therapist fails to see patients who have been assigned to him or her. This may sound insane, but it happens. It has been my experience that there are therapists who may do an initial assessment and then never see that patient again. Some would argue a patient does not need to be seen unless he or she calls for a follow-up appointment. It might be acceptable to not see a patient after an initial assessment if...

- a follow-up appointment was during the initial assessment and the patient didn't show up,
- the patient referred him or herself and then changed his or her mind,
- the patient chose another agency or therapist,
- the initial referral was totally inappropriate (however, some argue that a therapist should see a patient at least three times before closing the case in order to better assess the patient's needs).

Your state licensing board will have its own laundry list of ethical standards similar to those of the code described above, as well as the codes of licensed professional counselors, marriage and family therapists, social workers, physical and occupational therapists, chiropractors, massage therapists, etc. Some codes are much more elaborating then others. Many codes try to cover every base. If this was baseball, health care would never get to home plate because of all the bases a player would have touch in order to score a point, or make a net profit. What happened to "do no harm"?

CRT&O

Case Study

You are a licensed health care provider and have been working for your employer for a year. You decide that you have learned enough about starting up your own business in the metropolitan city where you now work. You have signed a contract with you employer that includes a non-compete clause, which says that you can open your own practice on the other side of town but you cannot in any way solicit patients you have seen with your employer and you cannot contact your current employer's referral sources for one year.

You find an office on the other side of town and decide to share it with two other health care providers. As you close your cases at your current employer several patients state that they wish to follow you to your new office. What do you tell them? Under what circumstances would you encourage them to see you at the other office? Would you be stealing or violating the non-compete clause in the contract you signed? What if you asked for the chance to bid against the employer in a contract with an organization that comes to you after you leave your employer? Is it ethical to submit a bid for the contract?

CRT&O

Business Ethics

A newspaper story told of the greed of the Chairman and Chief Executive of UnitedHealth Group, Inc. Dr. William McGuire, received over $94 million in total compensation, which represented an increase of 10 times what he made the previous year. UnitedHealth Inc. is reported to be the nation's largest services provider. Dr. McGuire's income "came from the exercise and sale of 1.9 million shares of UnitedHealth stock, which netted him $84.2 million."(7) His president and chief operation officer exercised 350,000 stock options and pocketed millions, too. Now the UnitedHealth may have to pay taxes on what they took. "The company has reported that the value realized from stock-options exercises by its five highest compensated executives, including CEO William McGuire, was $142.1 million in 2003, $191.5 million in 2004 and $12.2 million in 2005. The Securities and Exchange Commission is investigating stock options timings at UnitedHealth and several other companies. United Health has reported significant tax benefits from deducting stock options gains of its employees." (8) Perhaps these numbers might pale when compared to Enron's CEO's compensation prior to the federal government's intervention and investigation into his company's accounting and billing systems.

Keep in mind that this year most HMOs are raising health care premiums an average of 14 percent. Also keep in mind that the federal government reports that during the past two years over 60 million people were uninsured at least part of each year. It's just good business, some would argue. It's hard to get good people, others might say. But might one see a correlation between rising health insurance premiums and the way HMOs do business? It may be business and it may be legal, but is it ethical?

What is not heard much is a therapist who is hired as a full time employee or a part-time contract therapist and they receive referrals from the company or group to work. At some point they decide to tell the patients that they are leaving the group and ask if the patient wants to keep seeing them or someone else from the group. The patients are often confused and don't want to lose someone who they have seeing for some time. Then the therapist closes the case for the group and opens one for himself. This happens more than one might think. Since this is not a violation of any licensing board's ethical standards, the only recourse is to separate the therapist from the agency and/or sue for violation of contract. What about the psychiatrist who has a private practice but also owns a group mental health practice and refers all his cases to his own agency? There is a psychiatrist in San Antonio who actively tells patients who are referred to him from other agencies or therapists not to return to their therapist because he wants them to see the therapists at his clinic. He claims he has better treatment success with the patients if they can be seen at his clinic by therapists who work at his clinic. He refuses to prescribe medication for them if they do not see "his" therapists.

Ethics involves learning what is right or wrong. Some people believe doing "right" means following a code of ethics of the organization or the professional association they belong to. Some people believe that the right thing is based on a moral principle, while others believe that the right thing depends on the situation. In any case, the individual has to make their best judgment. Whether or not ethics is a "science of conduct" or not depends on what philosopher one reads or believes in; however, defining an ethical standard is a statement of a moral value of an individual. Business ethics is values management.

Business ethics is a term that attempts to describe behavior in the workplace. Training in business ethics informs employees at all levels of an organization of management's expectations for human interactions. Unfortunately, many training programs on ethics appear to be taken nonchalantly by many employees because they view standards of ethics as a simplistic statement of "Don't fight," "Don't lie," "Don't have sex in the office," "Don't steal," "Don't offend anyone," etc. Today most business schools provide some training in business ethics. They do this because there have been numerous employees and management personnel in corporate and government organizations and agencies who have taken part various criminal activities that have brought shame and embarrassment to their organizations. White collar crime in corporate America (i.e., Enron, WorldCom, Halliburton), in the media (i.e., Dan Rather of CBS News (who said there were certain documents that would embarrass President George W. Bush when there was no such documents, Jayson Blair former New York Times reporter for plagiarism, Globe magazine and England's Daily Mail for publication of false stories, Stephen Glass, writer with the New Republic for creating people, facts and events) or in the governmental hierarchy (i.e., Richard Nixon, Spiro Agnew, William Clinton), breaks down the trust, respect and confidence with the general public.

Business ethics can improve society's trust, respect and confidence in corporate America. Ethics training can be a good insurance policy to ensure that company policies and procedures are not only ethical but legal. It also is a good risk management factor because it can help avoid criminal acts of omission and may affect the level of fines that may or may not be accessed by a judicial authority.

Communications and the Healing Process

Communication is the use of words to exchange meanings. The patient is goes to the doctor or therapist for advice and guidance which leads to a decrease in symptomology and pain. It is essential for motivating the patient to want to get better and to comply with the suggestions of the doctor or therapist. Milton Erickson, M.D. and noted psychotherapist and hypnotherapist, was a master at helping patients reduce their fears and anxiety to increase their compliance with his treatment. Health care providers must come to realize whom they are really working for and should not abandon the patient-centered ethic that has grounded the health care profession. John Benson, M.D., served as the senior scholar with the Center for Ethics in Health Care during his tenure at Oregon Health & Science University. "Studies have demonstrated again and again the role that positive communication plays in health outcomes. Patients recover faster, feel less pain and stress, adhere better to their own treatment plans, and a have a higher level of overall satisfaction when good communication is part of their care." (9)

Telepsychotherapy

The practice of telepsychotherapy raises many interesting ethical and practical questions. To start, we must ask, "Is the telephone becoming a treatment tool?" Joyce Aronson, Ph.D., believes it is and she has edited a book, *Use of the Telephone in Psychotherapy*, and has made her own contribution to the book in support of this concept. "The increasing complexity of our social structure and consequently our patients' lives has resulted in an expanded use of the telephone in clinical work. Once confined to crisis situations, telephone contact now serves a multitude of therapeutic functions, and maintaining ongoing treatment when distance or other factors prevent in-person sessions is only one of them. The telephone can promote object constancy, provide a transitional space, or build a working alliance with the parents of child patients – and these are just some of the ways that it can enable and enhance the psychotherapeutic process." (10)

Face-to-face can lead to telephone therapy. A woman was treated by a therapist for 15 years, the first 3 years were face-to-face and the last 12 were by telephone. She reports that the patient agrees with her that "the ongoing treatment relationship has been life-sustaining for her – far outweighing whatever negative impact there might have been from the loss of face-to-face contact." (11)

The use of telepsychotherapy and telemedicine has been expanding with the advent of the Internet and videoconferencing. As a result new laws and guidelines have been discussed and are being implemented in many states. According to Sylvan Schafer, J.D., Ph.D., this rapid expansion has changed the legal landscape. The biggest fear is that "telepsychotherapy could lead to exploitation of the practitioners and force them to treat patients without face-to-face contact in order to reduce costs." (12)

"The rational for telepsychotherapy is that the process makes treatment available to patients who live in remote areas or who are unable to travel. This is especially useful for those who are disabled, phobic, or embarrassed to come in person. In addition, the process makes it possible for experts to provide consultations to other therapists. The telephone may also make it easier for psychotherapy patients to seek help, since it may remove some of the stigma and emotional inhibitions that prevent some potential patients from seeking face-to-face help." (13) "The issue of malpractice for telepsychotherapy involves fundamental questions about the nature of the psychodiagnostic and psychotherapeutic process." (14)

The use of telepsychotherapy or telemedicine or teleconferencing also raises questions of liability. Telepsychotherapy may be considered a "lesser form of psychotherapy and the therapist might be deemed to have practiced below the standard of the profession." (15) Then there is the question of privacy. It might not be clear that someone else is in the room with the patient providing some type of coaching, or just listening in on the conversation. The threats to privacy and confidentiality are both legal and technological. With the new HIPPA guidelines, it isn't clear how one can provide telemedicine, teleconferencing and psychotherapy and still meet HIPPA standards. Whenever something goes out across the Internet or airwaves there is a good chance that someone can intercept the transmission and listen in or watch the conversations. While there is a need to reduce costs of health care, much more needs to be done to protect privacy and confidentiality across telephone lines, the Internet, and the airwaves.

Biomedical Ethics

Biomedical ethics have changed greatly over the last five years. So many new developments have been made in research, and these affect all health care providers in one way or another. Health care providers need to have a working knowledge of these issues in order to be able to understand and work successfully with those patients who may be struggling with one of the following new issues:

- prenatal diagnosis of fetal disorders
- the role of the family in medical decision-making
- patient self-determination
- competency and assisted suicide
- institutionalization of chronic schizophrenics
- quality of life and long-term care
- research on the mentally disabled
- understanding or controlling AIDS
- care of people who are ill and hopeless
- problems with futility (treating diseases/disorders where there is no hope of getting better and may be terminal)
- stem cell research
- rationing health care
- social obligations of health care practitioners, and
- equality and inequity of health care. (14)

Domestic Violence

Having received my graduate training prior to 1980 I probably missed a course on how to understand, respond to and treat domestic violence. In supervising a number of therapists over the past ten years, I don't recall one who had a course on it, even though two of the therapists were licensed family and marriage therapists. In any case, the issues are complex and a serious health consequence for women and their children who witness it, and there are a number of hidden costs that need more light than darkness. Costs include financial, time away from families and work, and emotional costs to families, to their children, to police organizations, corporate America, to society, and to the energy of the therapists who accept these cases.

"Listening to women describe the violence in their lives can have a significant psychological impact on providers." (15) When health care workers, and especially psychotherapists and social workers, are not specifically trained to deal with psychological trauma, they are forced to go inward to rely on their own images and experiences and traumas. "Given the prevalence of violence against women in this society, a significant number of physicians will have experienced or witnessed abuse in their own lives. These issues touch too close to home for many health care providers, who may be understandably reluctant to have their own painful experiences evoked while trying to function in a professional capacity." (16) An ethical issue here is whether a provider in any health care discipline should be offering clinical services to someone who has similar experiences in his or her own life? Given the effects of stress of treating people who have had similar experiences in their lives, health care providers should probably refer out to other providers. The second ethical issue might be if we are not trained to treat a specific disorder, should we be trying to do therapy for that disorder?

Abortion and Gay Marriages

Can and should health care providers attempt to avoid difficult issues? Most therapists are pretty passionate individuals who have a sound rationale for their long-held beliefs and values. Having said that, can there be a middle ground and secondly, can the therapist enter the arena of therapy with a professional presentation rather than an accusatory one? Two issues that may evoke strong reactions and feelings in therapists are abortion and gay marriage. These issues are complex, have divided much of our country, and have caused much discomfort with those involved in this social debate.

Personally, when I am in the room with a woman who is considering an abortion or who has had one, the center of therapy is not the unborn, but the person sitting in front of me with her suitcase filled with guilt, fear, anxiety, depression, anger and pain. To me ignoring this woman and going instead to the baby are acts of abandonment and a betrayal of trust. Others may feel that, "since I'm a Christian I have a higher calling to help this lady return to her God and ask for forgiveness."

Identity issues can be difficult if one is shaky about his or her own identity. But when faced with a gay or lesbian couple, one quickly realizes, I hope, that they are human beings who have similar issues as heterosexual couples. Their preferences are different, their style of life and presentation are different, but they want love, sharing, caring, and to feel accepted and part of something bigger then themselves, and they are choosing to live their lives with a member of the same gender rather than the opposite sex. It took a long time before society was willing to accept, it may take longer to for mainstream America to accept the concept of a marriage for them. If your belief system will not accept this concept, can you be honest with the clients and exclude yourself as their therapist? Would it more or less ethical to refer them to a gay or lesbian therapist or to another therapist who has no problems working with them?

A middle road is not an invitation to compromise, and I'm not suggesting that we have to agree with our clients on every issue surrounding abortion or gay marriages. It means finding a common ground and discussing it, maybe finding ways to expand it. For these people, it means starting at a place where the patient(s) are and helping them find the pathway to where they want to be, not where you or I want to be. This is in many ways like working with other type of problems.

Self-Determination

Over 12 years ago the federal Patient Self-Determination Act (PSDA) became law. The PSDA requires Medicaid and Medicare institutional providers to do the following:

1. provide written information to in-patients upon admission (or upon enrollment or initial entry into service) about each of the following: the person's rights under law to make health care decisions,
2. including the right to accept or refuse treatment
3. the provider's written policies concerning implementation of those rights;
4. document in the person's medical record, whether or not the person has completed an advance directive;
5. ensure compliance with state laws concerning advance directives;
6. provide education for staff and the community. (17)

This act was passed in 1991 to recognize the rights of all patients. The Health Care Financing Administration created this act, which requires all health care facilities (one-person offices to groups to hospitals) that receive any federal funds, to tell all patients that they have a right to refuse treatment. This act requires a form that expresses these rights to a patient, and the patient should sign it to prove they read or were told of this right. Not only does this act reinforce the self-determination of patients, but it also provides another vehicle to document a patient's wishes in order to minimize the need for litigation.

An 82-year-old man entered an Ohio hospital for treatment of a coronary problem. Despite having a do-not-resuscitate (DNR) order, when he stopped breathing was resuscitated. Later, he suffered a stroke and was partially paralyzed and was sent to a long-term care facility. He sued the hospital for "wrongful life." Two years later he died. The case went to court, was appealed, and finally the Ohio Supreme Court dismissed the case. "It ruled that even though the hospital might be accused of committing a battery (legally defined as any uncontested touching, such as unrequested medical treatment), unless the plaintiff could show that the battery actually caused a further impairment such as the man's stroke and paralysis; there was no harm from treating a person against his wishes." (18)

PSDA is all about choice. In the 1990s the percentage of people who signed PSDAs was between 15 – 20 percent. People like choices; it's the American way. You don't go into your family grocery story and only find one choice of everything. That store would not be in business very long. Even when it comes to being medically resuscitated, it's a choice. But for emergency personnel and for physicians, having to pull back from resuscitation technically contradicts The Code. The question is, is it ethical to honor someone's wish not to be resuscitated, something that is required under the PSDA, and to do nothing to save a person from dying?

If people can refuse doctor suggested treatment for a tumor, or diabetes, or some other disorder or disease, can a paranoid schizophrenic refuse medication treatment? What are the ethical considerations for handling refusal of treatment for depression or other type of mental health illness? For children to be kept home from school by their parents after the child refuses to attend school, often child protective services are called and the parents are accused of child neglect (educational). Do providers (medical, chiropractic, social workers, etc., have the duty to report parents to child protective services for not sending their kids to school or not giving them the medication their primary care provider recommends? In Texas Medicaid is run by managed care organizations who report they have "case managers" who will respond to families who are refusing treatment from their providers (medical and mental health). This means that if they do not show up for an appointment the case manager can be called and they will call the patient or their family to inquiry and urge compliance. They also may be told that if the family refuses treatment or is non-compliant, they may lose their health insurance for that problem. Is this ethical and or legal?

In Corpus Christi a teenager was removed from her home because her family refused to continue her radiation therapy treatment for Hodgkin's disease. Child protective service lawyers asked a local court to remove the 13-year-old girl after she refused treatment and began eating foods that were not recommended by her doctors. "Officials from the Department of Family and Protective Services stepped in," accusing the family of medical neglect. A juvenile court judge stepped in and placed her in "temporary foster care and gave state officials the power to decide her course of treatment. Since then, the officials have been following the recommendations of doctors at M.D. Anderson"(Houston, TX). (19) This is not an isolated case. Paranoid Schizophrenics, when they go off their medications are normally placed by police officials under the directions of the patient's doctor in a psychiatric hospital included state hospitals. They are normally there are a week or two as they get back on their medications and "stabilize" allowing their doctors to discharge them again. Those with depression with suicidal ideations and gestures also are placed in psychiatric hospitals or wards until their ideations decrease. But have you ever heard about a patient with obsessive compulsive disorder, panic attacks, or attention deficit hyperactive disorder going off their medication and anyone placing them in a hospital or child protective services being called?

Or consider the case of a person that patient that is an auto accident and goes to a chiropractor who recommends treatment which he starts then stops when he started feeling better because he is afraid he'll be asked to return to work which he doesn't want to do until there is a settlement? Or the workers' compensation case where the patient is being treated by a physical therapist when the patient reports they can not continue because the pain is too great? The physical therapist will have to report the patient's condition and refusal to continue to the case manager of the case who may choose to close the case until the patient agrees to comply or until their benefits run out. These are all cases that may be considered non-compliant where the provider has to make a report of progress to the insurance company or case manager. What are the ethical implications in these cases?

Physician-Assisted Suicide

It difficult to talk about ethical issues in health care without discussing another controversial subject: assisted suicide. Subjects in ethics are seldom cut and dried or black and white. The whole concept of physician-assisted suicide is to allow those with a hopeless and chronic illness to make a final choice: when to die. Many consider this "mercy killing," others argue that people should be allowed to live and die with dignity. Although this group of individuals (who are suffering from chronic pain from a terminal illness) remains small in comparison to the overall population who are chronically sick, this group tends to suffer intolerably before death, despite the strongest of medicines. A few of these individuals would rather die then live any longer in this state, which torches their bodies and minds with unbelievable and unending pain and fear.

A few examples of this group of (terminally ill patients) individuals include "a former athlete, weighing 80 lb after an eight-year struggle with acquired immune deficiency syndrome (AIDS), who is losing his sight and his memory and is terrified of AIDS dementia; a mother of seven children, continually exhausted and bed-bound at home with a gaping, foul-smelling, open wound in her abdomen, who can no longer eat and who no longer wants to fight ovarian cancer; a fiercely independent retired factory worker, quadriplegic from amyotrophic lateral sclerosis, who no longer wants to linger in a helpless, dependent state waiting and hoping for death; a writer with extensive bone metastases from lung cancer that has not responded to chemotherapy or radiation, who cannot accept the daily choice he must make between sedation and severe pain; and a physician colleague, dying of respiratory failure from progressive pulmonary fibrosis, who does not want to be maintained on a ventilator but is equally terrified of suffocation." (20)

There are two ways that the patient's wish for death can come true. One is by physician-assisted suicide and the other is by voluntary euthanasia. The difference between these two choices is in the overall balance of power for either the doctor or the patient. In physician-assisted suicide the balance of power is more or less equal between doctor and patient. The final act is the patient's, and there is a reduced risk of coercion or abuse by the physician, family or friends. "The physician is counselor and witness and makes the means available, but ultimately the patient must be the one to act or not act. In voluntary euthanasia, the physician both provides the means and carries out the final act, with greatly amplified power over the patient and an increased risk of error, coercion or abuse." (21)

Physicians are placed into a situation that creates a moral dilemma. While they may feel sympathetic to the patient's condition and his or her desire to end it, there are laws forbidding assisting patients in their request for death. Various medical and legal groups have discussed these issues in an effort to propose clinical criteria for physician-assisted suicide. While such criterion has been proposed, there remains the balance of risks and benefits. It may very risky, in this managed care society, for licensed physicians to take a life. It is also argued that licensing physicians to take a life, no matter how noble the intent would destroy the identity of the medical profession and its central ethos, protecting the sanctity of life. Are there any circumstances where assisted suicide may be the only ethical action to take?

Managed Care (or Managed Costs or Managed Rights or Entitlements)

Since the advent of managed care new ethical and legal issues have emerged. Managed care has become known as "managed costs," and generally physicians and other health care providers have a different perspective on priorities in health care, one that is not centered on the cost of care but is instead concerned about producing the best outcomes for patients. Health care providers generally do all they can do for patients in order to improve their physical and mental health. Managed care has been accused of making decisions that impede quality service in order to save money. Where health care providers attempt to maximize health care, managed care is seen as attempting to minimize heath care delivery. Where as health care providers attempt to improve the relationship between themselves and their patients, managed care emphasizes spending less time with patients, and some would argue that the managed care industry interferes between doctor and patient.

Some have argued that managed care has destroyed the relationship between patient and provider by interfering with patients ability to choose their caregivers, by impending provider competence, by entering the patient-provider relationship and effecting changes in what is said and how it is said, by discouraging compassion, by interfering in a provider's efforts to create a continuity of care, and finally, by bringing a conflict of interest into the relationship. They argue that the increasing restrictions on providers threatens access to health care, limits the treatments and medications that can be offered or prescribed, limits the amount of sessions patients can be seen, and erodes the trust between provider and patient.

Managed care has offered physicians capitation incentives to reduce services. Capitation pays doctors x number of dollars for each patient under their plan each month, whether those patients are seen or not. Capitation encourages doctors to do less rather than more, while fee-for-services encourages doctors to do more for patients. No method of health care reimbursement is devoid of financial self-interest. This is because managed care organizations use "managers" who may or may not have much experience in health care delivery. These "managers" are loyal to their organizational goals of managing costs rather than managing disease and disorders. "In captivated managed care, and especially in global capitation, the doctor who takes home more does so by spending less on patients. With just this conflict in mind, the Health Care Financing Administration's new rules on incentives limit the amount of potential bonuses to 25 percent." (22)

"In particular, by creating conflicting loyalties for the physician, some of the techniques of managed care can undermine the physician's fundamental obligation to serve as the patient advocate. Moreover, in their zeal to control utilization, managed care plans may withhold authorizations for appropriate diagnostic procedures or treatment modalities from patients." (23)

Health care providers of all disciplines face these ethical dilemmas today as never before because state legislators have also endorsed the control concepts and precepts of managed care. During the past two years (2003-2004) various state legislators have been attempting to balance budgets by cutting social programs and health care benefits for thousands of children and adults. Mental health has been hit especially hard with reductions in States' Children Health Insurance Programs (SCHIPS) and Medicaid. In Texas adults can no longer receive psychotherapy if they have Medicaid. They can received a limited number of medical evaluations by psychiatrists, and only those with serious disorders (i.e., schizophrenia, bipolar, and major depression) can be seen by Community Mental Health and Mental Retardation Centers (MHMR). Normally there is a waiting list, and only a few of these patients may see a licensed therapist. Due to serious cuts in their funding, MHMR programs have become more restrictive and selective in whom they will treat.

Legislators excuse their decisions on a change of priorities. Today's mantra is "no new taxes," and legislators claim that their constitutions demand lower taxes, so they have no alternative. The consequences of these choices include a decreasing number of programs to meet the mental health needs. More adults are being jailed despite serious mental health problems. Juvenile residency (Youth Authority in Texas) programs report that a majority of their adolescents suffer from a number of mental health and substance abuse problems.

Another issue for physicians and therapists alike is when they spend more time explaining about the patients' HMO requirements, filling out different claim forms, collecting a co-payment, obtaining an authorization within the given time limit, etc....then treatment has become a secondary issue. Health care providers are expected to collect co-payments. If you do not collect these co-payments, the managed care organization company could contend that you are not in compliance with their policy and your contract with them and they can close the panel to you and ask for some money back. Getting "on" a panel means acceptance of your application which includes copies of your professional licenses, references and your professional liability policy.

HMOs, and now Medicare and Medicaid, provide formularies to doctors who prescribe medication. "The goal of a formulary, which is simply a list of approved medications, is to limit the use of expensive medicines, encouraging the cheaper, generic versions." (24) What happens when requests for more sessions or medical services are denied? Many health care providers are scared of "waking up the giant" by protesting a denied request so they may "punt," (a favorite term from football that means when you can't get your goal, you "punt" to the other team and hope other opportunities to "score" open up later) while others see an obligation to try and appeal the denial. Some providers may argue that we have an obligation to advocate for our patients. In a case where a patient was suing a state Medicaid plan for damages resulting from denial of care, the California Judge who heard the case wrote that "The physician who complies without protest with the limitations imposed by a third-party payer, when his medical judgment dictates otherwise, cannot avoid his ultimate responsibility for the patient's care.' "(25)

Many believe that HMOs and Medicaid and Medicare diminish mental health services by using a combination of policies (balancing the budget, no new taxes!) and by implementing procedures that make treatment inaccessible and/or undesirable. Several organizations have been forming to alert consumers of mental health services on ways to understand what role managed care plays and what you can do to get better services. Obtaining services through gate keeping, denying coverage, authorizing only a few sessions and asking for additional reports from the mental health professionals are just a few ways managed care controls how much health care you get. Some call it "invisible rationing." Mental health issues affect most people at some point in their lives. "However, in spite of the need for mental health services, mental health has been a primary target for managed-health-care cost cutting. Even though health insurance has historically restricted and under funded mental health services, since 1988 managed care has further reduced mental health coverage by eliminating 54% of insurance-based mental health funding. This cut in mental health funds is seven times as severe as the managed care cut in overall health care spending. Making matters worse, independent audits of managed mental health companies show that over 50% of mental health funds are now consumed by the administration and profit expenses created by managed care companies." (26)

What is the ethical way of dealing with a patient who has lost his or her mental health benefits? What is your legal or/and ethical obligation? Is it considered ethical to encourage your patients to begin writing letters of protest to their state representatives and senators? Should you write the letters to their MCO or HMO?

Social Policy

Do the citizens have a constitutional right to health care? Does it have to be quality health care? Does it have to include transplants? Does it have to include long-term care? Does it have to include quadruple bypass surgery, or a prosthesis, or dental work, or chiropractic treatments, or physical and occupational therapy, or acupuncture, or biofeedback or massage therapy? Does mental health care have to be provided?

Is there a social value to health care? Is health care worth the cost? Is one segment of health care worth the cost and another not worth it? When government cuts health care programs in order to balance the budget, is that insurance fraud?

Dual Relating and Dual Relationships

"In 1973 the American Psychological Association (APA), in an effort to curb a Pandora 's Box when it coined the term *dual relationship* in its Code of Ethics. Since then, every aspect of the psychotherapeutic relationship has been colored with continual concern, frustration, and doubt. The faulty shift of ethical focus from damaging exploitation to dual relationships has led to widespread misunderstanding and incessant moralizing that has undermined the spontaneous, creative and unique aspects of the personal relationships that are essential to the psychotherapeutic process. Dynamic and systems-oriented psychotherapies cannot be practiced without various forms of dual relating. But we have wrongly been told that dual relating is unethical." (27)

If you practice in the same area as you live you are likely to run into patients and their families. It may be at church, while shopping, at sporting events, at your child's school, and/or at the bank. While this can happen in a metropolitan community, it is much more common in a rural community. There can be events and situations that you may share with a patient and/or their family that might constitute dual relating but do not violate code of ethics under dual relationships. Dual relating refers to relating to a patient from different stances or roles, i.e., therapist, business partner, lover, spiritual leader, etc. Gradually professional associations and board of examiners are acknowledging this position.

Boundaries and boundary violations are carried into the therapeutic relationship. Some are expressed, some are withheld, some consciously, some not. These continuous mixing and merging then separate, only to re-merge later in the process of interactions between patient and psychotherapist. Boundaries are challenged and re-challenged in a therapeutic relationship as in the child-mother relationship.

Psychotherapists are change agents, whether as psychoanalysis, cognitive behavioralist, or reality therapist. In any therapy mode duality (dual relating) is an issue. So is the liability of not knowing the law or the code of ethics for the licensed professional. When insight is gained, sometimes it is painful. When images from the past are remembered they can be painful. When suicidal ideations are denied but appear later outside of therapy, often the therapist is accused of knowing about the threat or people say he or she "should have known" about the possibility of a suicidal threat or how the patient would react given some painful images. The idea that a therapist "**should have known**" lacks any responsible therapy research or even a single theoretical tract in the study of psychotherapy. However, it is an idea that is used in many arguments by attorneys or even association boards or state boards of examination for licensing professional therapists, psychologists or social workers.

While dual relating exists in transference (the patient transferring to the therapist or seeing the therapist as their father or mother, etc.) counter-transference (the therapist transferring their feelings onto the patient as if the patience has the same feelings the therapist is having), resistance and interpretation, it can be a powerful tool for creating motion in the transformation process. Here are a few suggestions for safeguarding against abuse while honoring the dual relating inherent in the practice of psychotherapy:

1. When any direct or indirect contact outside the formal therapeutic setting exists between therapist and client, a consultant or third-party case monitor should be sought at regular intervals to evaluate and comment on the course of therapy.

2. To protect privacy and confidentiality, all appearances of a dual relationship that might potentially be seen by third parties and

conceivably be reported to boards and committees for open investigation should be avoided.

3. An alternative approach is for the therapist to have recourse to settling the dispute in civil court, where full discovery and due process are guaranteed, as they are not under administrative law, and where malpractice insurance serves to protect the therapist from frivolous accusations that licensing boards are famous for prosecuting. We know that ethics committees and governing boards are prey to political and economic pressures and various pre-established biases, so that a therapist acting in good faith and upon sound professional opinion is not assured of a fair judgment. (28)

Confidentiality

In the chapter on legal liabilities we discussed how HIPPA was created in large part due to the need to reinforce patient confidentiality. Too many patients walk into an office and the clerk or nurse discusses why they are there. This is often done in front of everyone in the reception room. Confidentiality is mentioned in this chapter on ethics because being sensitive to the needs of a patient is an ethical issue. Protecting these rights is also an ethical issue. Helping the patient understand the reasons for therapy, how the treatment process works, and with whom information may be shared with and why are ethical AND legal obligations.

"Patient confidentiality remains one of the sacrosanct and leading ideas in the time-honored Hippocratic Oath. As a general rule, information between healthcare professionals and the patient must remain confidential and can be shared with others only if medically necessary or legally mandated. For instance, it is legally required for physicians to report gunshot wounds and instances of child abuse.

Physicians are also required to report to the proper authority's medical conditions that adversely affect the safety of society, such as a heart condition of a flight controller." (29)

Psychologists, social workers and all mental health professionals have similar obligations. When working with a referral from the local Child Protective Service (CPS), patients are required to be told about what information the professional will disclose to CPS as well as the primary physician and/or any other medical or mental health professional. In addition, all patients need to be told how you will deal with information regarding child abuse or neglect, suicidal ideas and gestures, and adult abuse or neglect.

Power Point

This chapter reviewed a number of ethical potholes that can trip a provider and cause one to fall on one's face. How you handle these situations can cause you to drop out of the profession or allow you to get up and, dust off the dirt and mud, and nurse your bruises back to heal as you continue your journey as a professional provider.

End of Chapter Review

Multiple Choice Questions:

1. How can the use of the telephone enable and enhance the psychotherapeutic process?
    a. It can promote object constancy
    b. It can provide a transitional space
    c. It can build a working alliance with the parents of child patients
    d. None of the above

2. Most Codes of Ethics admonish about:
    a. Any misleading, deceptive, fraudulent or exaggerated claim or statement about their license
    b. Making any misleading statement about their background or training, experience or education or professional affiliations
    c. Making false statements about their fees or publications
    d. Making any promise of "healing or curing" the patient
    e. All the above
    f. A, B, C

3. Managed care has become known as:
    a. An industry that attempts to impair access to health care
    b. An industry that destroys health care
    c. Managed costs
    d. A road block to quality care

4. Which of the following is NOT one of the four benchmarks of Principlism:
    a. Beneficence
    b. Nonmaleficence
    c. Autonomy
    d. Equality

5. The Patient Self-Determination Act (PSDA) is about:

a. Justice
b. Fairness
c. Ethics
d. Choice

Rethink Questions:

1. As a health care provider, under what circumstances can you turn down a patient?
2. White collar crimes bring questions about how an organization can deal with executives who are alleged to have committed a crime or who has done something that embarrasses the organization. Discuss what choices the organization has at this point.
3. Should the purpose and policies of professional boards be changed to reflect the ethical issues of today?
4. Discuss ways to protect one's practice from over-zealous social workers at CPS and should these unlicensed workers have some type of license or/and professional liability?
5. Explain how better communications between health care provider and patient affects the motivation and health of the patient.

Personal Observation Exercise

Go to the Oregon Health & Science University website and look up the Center for Ethics in Health Care. Be prepared to discuss their curriculum and how it helps doctors "be better doctors".

References

1. Texas Administrative Code of Ethics, 1990.
2. Ibid
3. Ibid

4. Ibid, p.2

5. Ibid. pp. 2 - 7

6. American Association of Marriage and Family Therapists, July 2001 to present, www.aamft.org/resources/LRMPlan/Ethics/ethicscode2001.asp

7. Smith, Scott D., UnitedHealth heads cash-in stock options, Minneapolis/St. Paul Business Journal, December 31, 2001, www.twincities.bizjournal.com/twincities/stories/2001/12/10/daily38.html

8. Wilbert, Lauren, Report: UnitedHealth may owe back taxes on stock options, Minneapolis/St. Paul Business Journal, *April 24, 2006,* www.bizjournals.com/twincities/stories/2006/04/24/daily62.html

9. Benson, John, M.D., **Focus on Ethics**, Center for Ethics in Health Care, University of Oregon, Spring 2004, p. 4.

10. Aronson, Joyce K., Ph.D., **Use of the Telephone in Psychotherapy**, p. xxi, Jason Aronson, Inc., Northvale, New Jersey, 2000.

11. Plummer, Jane and Martha Stark, Long-Term Therapy by Telephone, p. 109, **Use of the Telephone in Psychotherapy**, Joyce Aronson, Editor, Jason Aronson, Inc., Northale, New Jersey, 2000.

12. Schaffer, Sylvan Legal and Ethical Issues, p.444, **Use of the Telephone in Psychotherapy**, Joyce Aronson, Editor, Jason Aronson, Inc., Northvale, New Jersey, 2000.

13. Ibid, p. 444.

14. Ibid, p. 445.

15. Monagle, John F. and David C. Thomasma, Eds., **Health Care Ethics**, pp. v-xiv, Aspen Publishers, Inc., Gaithersburg, Maryland, 1998.

16. Warshaw, Carole, <u>Domestic Violence: Changing Theory, Changing</u> Practice, p. 129, **Health Care Ethics,** John F. Monagle and David C. Thomasma, Eds., Aspen Publishers, Inc., Gaithersburg, Maryland, 1998.

17. Ibid.

18. Clarke, David B., <u>The Patient Self-Determination</u> Act, p. 92, **Health Care Ethics,** John F. Monagle and David C. Thomasma, Eds., Aspen Publishers, Inc., Gaithersburg, Maryland, 1998.

19. Ibid, p. 111.

20. Caller-Times, Scripps Texas, L.P., Corpus Christi, TX pp. 1A and 8A, October 29, 2005.

21. Quill, Thomas, Christine K. Cassel and Diane E. Meier, <u>Care of the Homelessly Ill: Proposed Clinical Critereia for Physician-Assisted Suicide</u>, p. 295, **Health Care Ethics,** John F. Monagle and David C. Thomasma, Eds., Aspen Publishers, Inc., Gaithersburg, Maryland, 1998.

22. Ibid, p. 296.

23. Tuckfelt, Sondra, Jeri Fink, and Muriel Prince Warren, **The Psychotherapists' Guide to Managed Care in the 21st Century**, p. 47, Jason Aronson, Inc., Northvale, New Jersey, 1997.

24. Ibid, p.48.

25. La Puma, John, M.D. <u>Should Capitation's Financial Incentives Be Part of Informed Consent to Treatment?,</u> Managed Care Magazine, April 1996, <u>www.managedcaremag.com/archives/9604/MC9604.ethics.shtml</u>

26. Miller, Ivan, <u>Mental Health Consumer Protection Manual</u>, National Coalition of Mental Health Professionals and Consumers, 4/29/06, <u>www.nomanagedcare.org/consum.html</u>

27. Hedges, Lawrence E., Ph.D., **Facing The Challenge Of**

Liability In Psychotherapy, Pp.113-114

28. Ibid, pp.127-130.

29. Brannigan, Michael C. and Judith A. Boss, <u>The Relationship Between Healthcare Professionals and Patients,</u> **Healthcare Ethics in a Diverse Society**, Mayfield Publishing Company, Mountain View, California, 2001, p.128

Chapter Four
Managing Outside Agitators

Summary

Today we have a crisis of values, of priorities, of passion and of work ethics. We have seen an erosion of our practices and our energy to practice, of companies that do not care, and of governmental agencies that act as if they want us to close and just go away. Cities and counties are putting mental health patients in jail and not treating them. State Hospitals are full and psychiatric patient beds are at a premium. Hospitals are fighting with states for reimbursement for indigent care, especially in the emergency rooms, that has increased in large part to lost jobs or small businesses that cannot afford health care insurance. All these problems are needs to be met and solved. They are created, in large part by the policies handled down from the White House to Congress to the agency bureaucrats to the State legislators to MCOs and HMOs to the general public. The problem went up with a load of similar problems and a few solutions and comes back down the laundry shoot looking like something else. In this chapter we will discuss these issues within the perimeters of public policy. We will also discuss how these polices address certain social values and political realities and how they effect both the provider and the patient.

You will learn in this chapter:

1. How people and organizations you don't know have an impact on your practice.

2. Where you can get information about some of these people

and organizations.

3. The importance of entitlement in the discussion of health care financing.

4. Why costs are not as high if you factor in the values of the services, including prevention.

5. The value of reforming alternatives to our present system of health care administration and delivery.

Public Policy

The word "politics" refers to the science of government; that part of government that regulates a state or nation. This regulates the preservation of the states' or nation's safety, peace, and prosperity, and for the improvement of the citizens' moral. The word "therapy" refers to the medical science of discovering, diagnosis, and creating remedies for diseases and disorders.

Since we are talking about the politics of therapy we can include the term "policy," since it is the engine that runs the politics of change, of direction, of power. Policy is a little harder to define crisply, lending itself to more of a comic relief. For example, Mark Twain wrote, "Honesty is the best policy when there is money in it." And Lyndon B. Johnson was quoted as saying, "It is common failing of totalitarian regimes that they cannot really understand the nature of our democracy. They mistake dissent for disloyalty. They mistake restlessness for a rejection of policy. They mistake a few committees for a county. They misjudge individual speeches for public policy." Former presidential candidate John Kerry was quoted as saying, "John Dean has "no" as a policy. 'No' is not a policy." Former presidential advisor Richard Allan is quoted as saying, "The transition team plans for policy review, prospective policy changes and the insertion of key personnel at the upper levels of government." We will be defining "policy" as any stated recommendations for direction of health care management, administration, delivery or financing. A policy is defined here as a recommendation, or a stated priority or statement presented as a policy that comes down from the federal or state government, from Think Tanks or Foundations or associations or special commissions or committees that have an impact on the legislations that affect health care in any way.

There are three criteria that must be met before an issue can be considered by policy makers:

- The specific issue must be the subject of widespread attention;
- A sizable proportion of the public must demand action;
- The issue must be the concern of an appropriate governmental unit. (1)

There are several liabilities that are created by these policies, some costly consequences. Those who sit on appointed policy making committees and commissions are considered, within the context of this chapter, as outside agitators since their decisions and policies effect the boundaries of our practices. They are not invited to our practices nor do they ask for our opinions. They may not have any experience in the delivery of health care nor in the development and management of a health care practice. However their decisions and policies along with their "hidden agendas" affect the development, administration, delivery, financing, and management of our hospitals, groups and private practices.

The purpose of this chapter is to discuss the implications of having our offices invaded by outsiders who serve as agitators. For example, managed care has been an appalling failure in its marketed goal of saving health care money. Yet they go on and on and on without regard of the tragedy they leave behind for patients as well as providers. They agitate in our fields of action without risking their own work environment, dictating our future without giving any consideration of how it may affect our practices. They are agitators in the sense that they tax our time, our energy, and our practices without asking how these changes will affect our practice. Their concern is not for our practices; it is for their positions in the governmental bureaucracy or in their managed care organization, in a Think Tank, or in the public's eye. They speak and they expect compliance. They don't even ask for understanding, only compliance. They don't bargain or give us additional resources to handle their policy which forces us to add people and time to comply. This amounts to taxation without representation.

Our business of healing was not always a business. It focused on developing clinical skills and techniques to help people gain greater insight, make better choices, develop an awareness of the consequences of their behaviors and, perhaps, have the time to help them find meaning and clarity. At one time our healing arts were respected, though not very well understood.

Health care has taken the blame for "rising health care costs." Providers are blamed for this problem due to errors in surgery and over billing and over servicing patients. Managed care has promised to take care of these problems by denying access, lowering reimbursement rates to providers, and increasing paper work and audits. They have all the leverage, and providers have little. While MCO CEOs take millions and billions to their banks, patients lose services and providers lose practices.

Most public policies began as little personal ones. As individuals understand and develop an argument for sharing their problem with others, questions began to shape and side issues and factors to be considered are discovered. The problem no longer belongs to one person or group as people began talking about it. As the problem shapes into focus and into a message, that others can understand and contribute to, slowly it moves into the media and more public exposure which leads to a wider discussion. At some point political candidate may choose to champion or at least float it out further into the sea of public opinion for more discussion and debate. Then a poll is taken and published.

Another way that public policy can take off fast is when there is a natural disaster or a terrorist attack on a community or state, such as four hurricanes in 2004 in Florida, the 911 attack in New York, or Hurricane Katrina in New Orleans, Mississippi and Alabama, August 2005.. Now the subject jumps out at the whole nation from the television and radio news programs and from the print media. We are glued to the horrific scenes as if we can not pull ourselves away from it. Congress members join the chorus of voices calling for some governmental intervention, i.e. the Federal emergency management agency, FEMA. Soon politicians are swarming the area getting their pictures taken, getting a lot of newsprint and television time. Money is promised to fix this and that and to "take care of the people". These are some of the same people who the previous week needed health care and couldn't get so have to stay sick or home from work. These are some of the same people who needed a job and couldn't find one for the past two years. These are some of the same people that needed medication but couldn't afford it or who were going bankrupt because their medical bills were not covered in total by their group or individual insurance. These issues reach the desks of those who sit in corporate or foundation "think tanks" and discuss "public policy". Decisions are made to search the literature, maybe commission a survey, do a two-year study and write some articles, maybe even a book.

Public policy issues have "windows of opportunity" that open and close in a fairly short period of time. Remember the bomb shelters that were built during the 50's? Or the Community Action Programs of the Johnson years? Gore's lock box or President Bush's alternative to Social Security? The environment issues are what people can argue about for years but it only stays in the forefront of the news media for much less time. For example, the issue of a warming climate is questioned and debated but not every night. Debates in public tend to come and go based upon increased temperatures in the summer, the ice glades melting, or severe changes in weather patterns.

When the legislators raise taxes on property, such as a house or business, to pay an increase in teachers' salaries, education administrators and school boards might be attacked by angry parents who report that the community is not getting their money's worth anyway, now they don't want to pay more. Crisis triggers crisis and chaos.

Triggers in health care include when the ERs are full, State Hospital beds are full, providers dropping contracts with certain MCOs, and the lost of health insurance or/and a job. Triggers in the economy may be an increase in unemployment, loss of jobs due to FAHFA or CAHFA, a high interest rate, or some natural disaster like a drought or a recession or inflation. "In the context of the political process, a triggering mechanism is a critical event (or set of events) that converts a routine problem into a widely shared, negative public response. This public response, in turn, is the basis for the policy issue that ensues in the wake of the triggering event. When an occurrence crystallizes a negative condition into a pressing political demand for change, the metamorphosis happens because of the staying power of the triggering mechanism." (2)

While many issues are extremely complex, others are more of a "crowd pleaser" like cutting taxes. Currently most state legislators are singing the song of "no new taxes". Thus when there are budget restrictions then the legislators have the task of picking which services to cut. Often they increase various fees and cut program. Most of the programs are social programs like entitlements such as Medicaid and welfare. This has caused an outcry from various groups but the outcry has not been loud enough or long enough to make a difference. When and only when legislators are thrown out of office and the reason given by exit polls is the cuts in social programs, and then nothing will change. Politians will assume that the people want to continue with "no new taxes" and with that is the loss to programs that do not seem to affect the majority of voters. Elected officers maintain power as long as they are re-elected while bureaucrats tend to get lost in the crowd and have a job for a much longer period of time. These are the people that often write changes or amendments into proposed legislation. This has increased the influence these people have on social and economic policies while remaining "hidden" for the most part from scrutiny and accountability.

Policies are used by politicians to garner votes and to rally certain populations that favor these policies. Some use media events, some use programmed public affair meetings such as "town hall" meetings, and others like Rick Perry, the Republican Governor of Texas, uses ministers to organize and drive their flocks to the voting booths. "Each briefing will provide important information and resources you can use in your own congregations to promote voting in Texas," reads one of the invitations. (3) The article also suggests that the Texas Restoration Project has been organized to help pastors mobilize their flocks behind the issues the Governor supports (against gay marriages, to re-elect Perry, etc.).

"To the most casual observer, these events are really campaign events," charged Dan Quinn, spokesperson for the Texas Freedom Network. But, according to the Rev. Laurence White, Our Savior Lutheran Church in Houston, "if anything, the political discussion has intruded into the life of the church in recent years as it has focused more and more on fundamental issues like the sanctity of life, marriage – things pastors have been preaching about for 2,000 years." (4)

When added up health care providers are a community and a community normally is interested in preserving its own sense of order and fair play. Most communities have an interest in some form of governing or management process and some means for resolving conflicts and challenges to the community and the community interests. Since health care providers are normally turf conscious, there have been limitations to their abilities to fight back. Members of the health care industry have been both confused and frustrated at their inability to stand up against those who would challenge their value and purpose by imposing non-health care management techniques on health care providers, like the management by leverage. (5) For example health care providers tend to believe that family practice physicians should be gatekeepers to health care but managed care organizations argue that this is antithetical to the survival of our economy and is likely to destroy the national budget. Both sides aggress that community survival, i.e. national survival, is important if we are going to be able to work and live within that community. "There is virtually never full agreement on the public interest, yet we need to make it a defining characteristic of the polis because so much of politics is people fighting over what the public interest is and trying to realize their own definitions of it." (6)

Healthy People 2010

A number of years ago the federal government put a committee together, through the Secretary of Health and Human Services, to study the health needs of Americans and to promote healthy people. In 1995 President Clinton signed the Healthy People 2000 bill and in 2000 President Bush signed in the Healthy People 2010 bill which provided the guidelines for an increase in the quality of life of people from birth to their grave. The committee that wrote this policy statement wrote it to promote and encourages state agencies and local communities to create action on health care issues. The federal government has also set aside funding for certain targeted projects.

The goals of Healthy People 2010 include:

- "Help individuals of all ages to increase life expectancy and improve their quality of life." At the beginning of the 20th century the life expectancy of a baby was 47.3 years. Today, the average life expectancy is over 77 years. This issue presents a new challenge to all health care providers, insurance companies, and the federal health programs (Medicare and Medicaid). Never, in the history of America, have there been so many people over the age of 65. These are the years where the greatest amount of health care is needed and where the costs are the greatest for a specific population.

- To eliminate health disparities among different segments of the population, including differences that occur between gender, race, ethnicity, education, income, disabilities, geographic location and sexual orientation.

Health care disparities continue to remain a problem in America. One is for the elderly who may have Medicare but who can not buy the medications their doctors prescribe because they live on fixed incomes. Hispanics and those living in poverty are not systematically forced off Medicaid due to "budget priorities". Foundations who provide grants to non-profit organizations follow the priorities of the government and fail to meet the needs of these people (i.e. rural and border communities). "Decades of studies that racial and ethnic minorities, in comparison with white people, suffer higher rates of diabetes, heart disease and HIV/AIDS, and African-Americans have shorter life expectancies and higher rates of infant mortality. In March 2002, the Institute of Medicine published a report highlighting several possible reasons. It said doctors and hospitals are always under pressure to save money and that cost savings may come at the expense of patients least educated about their treatment options and least likely to push their doctor for more services. This is particularly true, the report said, for patients who are not native English speakers." (7)

Midway through the second 10 year-year evidence-based health objectives for improving the health of Americans, there is a process of assessing the progress of the objectives and the data trends. Public comments have been invited by the general public from August 15, 2005 through September 15, 2005. The Healthy People program is managed by the Office of Disease Prevention and Health Promotion, U. S. Department of Health and Human Services. (8)

In the June 19, 2004 issue of the British Medical Journal (BMJ) it was reported that President George Bush was planning to propose screening the whole U.S. population for mental illness. While the primary goal of the President's New Freedom Commission on Mental Health is to integrate mentally ill patients fully into the community, it goes much farther by recommending comprehensive mental-health screening for "consumers of all ages," including preschool children. The Commission established a number of goals and recommendations to include early mental health screening, assessment, and referral to services. Other goals included the establishment of electronic medical records for mental health purposes. What the Commission DID NOT provide for was the supervision of the screeners. Therefore, the results of the screening may be distorted by individual biases, influences of culture, religion and political agendas. (9)   While this program stems from well-meaning suggestions, it is built on a stack of public governmental departments each with numerous Secretaries and Assistant Secretaries and Deputy Secretaries and Administrators with another list of Senior Assistant Administrators, etc. "The fastest spreading titles continue to be alter-ego deputies, including chiefs of staff to secretaries, deputy secretaries, under secretaries, deputy secretaries, assistant secretaries, deputy assistant secretaries, associate deputy assistant secretaries, associate assistant secretaries, administrators, deputy administrators, associate administrators, and assistant administrators. Bluntly put, having a chief of staff has become a signal of one's importance in the bureaucratic pecking order. Chiefs of staff are not mere minions-their job descriptions usually include de facto supervisory responsibilities within their units, and they often act as gatekeepers for their principal. Although many of these titles exist in only one or two departments, past experience suggests that they will spread quickly – the first chief of staff to a secretary was created in 1981, spread to 10 additional departments by 1992, and now exists in 14 of 15." (10)

Health care providers provide health care. Administrators administrate programs but do not have the knowledge, the degree or license, to help and heal the sick. If the administrators think health care providers make too much money, why are they not in medical school? If health care is of value, is the delivery of health care of less value then the administration and financing of health care? With multi-levels of government and of managed care, the actual delivery of health care has been pushed further and further back on the agenda of priorities. The administrators have stolen the money from the providers and have stored it in their own pockets and mattresses. The U. S. Attorney General should investigate these agencies and organizations for health care fraud! America's leaders have their priorities upside down. It's time for health care providers to speak-out more in the media, in public, stressing what health care can do and not about who can or can not access health care and blaming the providers for the costs of health care. It's time for the public to get re-educated about the value of health care in their lives, not just the emergency care, but the preventive services, and not just the physical medical care but also how mental health services can improve the quality and quantity of life.

An Expanding Industry

"Health care in the United States now is a $1.7 trillion industry, encompassing significant portions of federal, state and local budgets, as well as a huge private sector market. The issues of growth, inflation, prices, sources of funding, as well as coverage and quality of services are central too much of today's health policy discussion." (11)

"Connecticut pays $626 million a year to health maintenance organizations that provide care for needy families, but state officials are fighting a request to let taxpayers know how that money is spent. The dispute began when a group of New Haven clinics noticed that their patients were having trouble getting appointments with private cardiologists and gastroenterologists to treat heart or digestive problems. Clinic operators suspected that the HMOs were paying such low rates for their patients covered by Medicaid that private doctors would not accept them." (12)

The Texas Department of Protective and Regulatory Services (TDPRS) has documented that 82% of the children in custody of that agency under parental relinquishment criteria are there because parents had no other way to access mental health services. There were 244 children relinquished in this last resort for mental health care category in 2002. With an average cost of $109.38 per day, these 244 children will cost the State $9.7 million for a year of care as compared to $6.3 million for community-based services. Often it is less than this if services are provided by non-MHMR providers who depend on Medicaid as a reimbursement rather than State grants like MHMR programs. Secondly, a majority of MHMR counselors or service providers are none licensed individuals who are trained to do their jobs by MHMR which uses grants to train them. Health care providers who are independent of MHMR receive no such training or grants but are licensed and have obtained graduate degrees and tend to have more therapy experience then many of those who work within MHMR. States cannot afford, in the long-run, to under-fund mental health services.

Loss of Competence

The Federal government has problems with the work ethics of employees like any other employer. Employees who are passive aggressive or who do not appreciate how valuable their tasks are to a department or company and how much others depend on them. According to a study by L. R. Huntoon, a practicing neurologist and editor-in-chief of the Journal of American Physicians and Surgeons, reports that customer service representatives gave the wrong answer 96 percent of the time. In comparison, Huntoon asked a toad a series of Medicare policy questions. The toad jumped right for "yes" and left for "no". The toad jumped in the right direction 50 percent of the time, a much more accurate rate then the customer service representatives! In 2003, Medicare received a total of 21 million "provider" inquiries; of those 21 million, Medicare's error rate would translate to 20,160,000 wrong answers. GAO (General Accounting Office) estimates that 500,000 of the 21 million were policy-oriented; overall, between 480,000 and 20,160,000 Medicare claims are incorrectly denied due to the incorrect information provided by Medicare representatives. With no accurate definition of accurate, it appears that CMS (Centers for Medicare and Medicaid Services) considers accuracy and competence to be irrelevant, says Huntoon. Dr. Huntoon also points out that Medicaid is the fastest growing expenses in all state budgets and that the National Governors Association in

December 2004 predicted that Medicaid is rapidly reaching a breaking point. (13)

Technocrats Taking Over

Ever since managed care organizations started influencing the practice of health care they have been increasing their control of costs by denying reimbursements for certain procedures, the number of sessions of psychotherapy, denying sessions without pre-approval, building filters to access, knocking providers off of their panels, cutting reimbursement rates to providers, and creating evidenced-based medicine. Providers of every discipline have expressed hesitance and reservations.

"The public needs to understand that evidence-based medicine (EBM) is an attack on the patient-doctor relationship. EBM is not individualized care. It is group-think medicine," says Twila Brase, president of Citizens' Council On Health Care (CCHC) and author of the report "How Technocrats are Taking Over the Practice of Medicine: A Wake-Up Call to the American People". (14)

The CCHC has expressed concern over the control MCOs and HMOs have over health care professionals. The concerns can be summarized in five points:

1. EBM is managed care no matter what the name it's still the same.

2. Science is not the basis of EBM despite what managed care organizations claim. In research there are subjective choices that are made which help form the "evidence" of EBM.

3. The guidelines of EBM are seen as outdated and in conflict with one another, biased, and single-deceased focused and the lack of individualization.

4. Under EBM practice guidelines come with mandated treatment. The organizations use computer programs to

monitor compliance and find ways to penalize providers who do not comply with their rules.

5. Providers complain that patients can be harmed by these rules and guidelines. They often join with those in England who have reported that the guidelines are used to implement health care rationing. (14)

The legislators that vote for laws often have very little background or knowledge on the subject they are voting on so they must depend on "experts" from their community or from their staff. Some effort has been made to provide legislators with the background knowledge needed the Networks Financial Institute at Indiana State University have developed an ongoing program to provide legislators from around the country and their staffs with the knowledge they need to set policies that meet the needs of the modern economy. They have established a curriculum of 15 courses that focus on the areas of market principles, supervision and regulation, product lines, company operations, and current topics in financial services. (15) They do not offer any health care courses.

Another problem is the lack of awareness of how valuable mental health services can be and ho much it can save in community expenditures. According to the Criminal Justice/Mental Health Consensus Project in the course of one year a person who has been repeatedly jailed, hospitalized, or admitted to detoxification centers can cost the State an estimated $55,000 each. Community-based services can reduce recidivism and close the revolving door, but authorities apparently do not know this or do not understand it, or choose to ignore this information. (16)

People with mental illness tend to serve longer prison sentences and recidivate at a higher rate then other inmates. Seventy-nine percent of local jail inmates with mental illness had prior criminal convictions compared to 71.6% of other inmates. (17) "The cost to Texas for 'revolving door offenders' is an estimated $682 million per year as compared to $92 million for treatment in a community mental health center." (18) "The mental health service is highly fragmented. Many who seek treatment are bewildered by the maze of paths into treatment, while others are stymied by lack of information about where to seek effective and affordable services. The juvenile justice system represents another pathway, although many overburdened facilities lack the staff required to deal with the magnitude of the mental health problems encountered. Of equal concern is whether the adult criminal justice and corrections systems, which encounter substantial numbers of detainees with mental illness, are equipped to handle these problems. Individuals with mental disorders often are neglected or victimized in these institutions." (19) People with mental illnesses are more likely to be victims rather than perpetrators of violence, inside or outside the criminal justice system. States like Texas outsource their prisons to contractors who operate all the programs in the prison including physical and mental health care. To Texas and Texas rural communities this system is operates as a "cash cow" generating millions for local and state agencies.

Accessibility

One of the needs is accessibility and at a lower cost. If there are ten therapists in each county the likelihood of the population receiving appropriate mental health care is significantly greater than if there was only one or none as there is in numerous rural communities. The more people that can deliver health care, the more patients that will receive it. Therefore, by basic mathematics health care dollars increase as more people go to a clinic or office to receive some type of health care. It increases as populations grow older. It increases every time someone is born. It increases as various deadly viruses spread through communities.

Politicians do not want to make decisions as to accessibility. They want someone else to be blamed by their communities for the lack of accessibility. State legislatures often develop voting systems that do not pinpoint each vote cast by each legislature. The State Representatives and State Senators from each district want their people to receive not only health care but superior health care. Secondly, they outsource the administration of Medicaid and who create a maze of companies that only deal with parts of the puzzle, such as traditional Medicaid, SCHIP's Medicaid, eligibility, claims, audits, R&Ss, payments, computer programs, credentialing, provider relations, and administration.

Legislators that represent rural communities are often out-voted and out-spent when it comes to political pressure in campaigns and in negotiations and trade-offs. Programs that restrict access include budget cuts, limiting Medicaid guarantees, limiting ways for individuals and families to sign-up and to qualify, spending caps, and not accepting or applying for matching federal funds.

Entitlements

Entitlements support accessibility. The discussion of funding for health care has become a basic issue and a moralistic question: Is everyone entitled, or has a right, to any health care service? To basic health care, top shelf, or some other type and quality of health care in the middle? And who or what determines that entitlement?

There are a number of entitlement programs supported by state and federal governments. Social Security, Medicare and Medicaid are a few. At this time any person who meets the criteria becomes eligibility established by each entitlement program. States are entitled to receive funds from the federal government for their pledged share of the costs of the program.

"Financing is fundamental to an entitlement program, because the financing structure must back up the legal obligation that the program creates. State and federal Medicaid funding is based on need, not on fixed budget, and this is what makes the entitlement to individuals possible. It means that all individuals within a state who meet Medicaid eligibility requirements can receive all of the services that state covers." (20)

Spending is determined by the number of people who use the services. They may use the medical services one year and no mental health benefits but in a few years they may use both types of services. None of these factors are fixed, number of services used, number of people using them are out of the control of state personnel. However, there are some ways they can affect the accessibility of patients: hiring managed care organizations to handle the administrative process. If you let the fox MCOs) guard the chickens (providers) you will have less providers. When you have less providers or when the state legislators cut access or entitlements, there are more people looking for alternative health care.

If you don't have insurance you don't go to the doctor unless there is an emergency and then you may choose to go the local Emergency Room. The costs are higher in the ER and you will pay more than those who have insurance (as noted in recent legal actions against hospitals). But will it be higher than if you had paid for an insurance policy for an entire year? If you go into the ER once a year, and it costs you $600 plus $150 in medicine, then your yearly costs are $750. Compare that to paying $350 per month or over $4200 per year. However, if you have to have surgery that costs $15,000 plus rehabilitation and medications, your insurance costs are probably over $20,000 which makes the insurance policy look pretty good. States think the same way. They have to find some way to hedge their risks and financial liability. States need a way to respond to these uncertainties. A preset amount of money set aside for all services, or divided among different type of services, might create an overestimate or an underestimate. An underestimate would lead to an unpleasant consequence: not being able to fund services to people who are entitled to them. They may only have $17,000,000 for the entire fiscal year for all health care benefits, so they find others who will share the risks. They provide contracts to managed care organizations that do the administrative work for part of the pie. For example, some will only see mental health patients, some only Medicaid SCHIPS program, some medical care only, etc.

When the states turn over the administrative controls to managed care organizations (MCO) they are affecting accessibility. Accessibility is a way to control the use of benefits. States will tell you that they turn to MCOs for administrative expertise and in an effort to lower costs. While there may be a glimmer of truth to this practice, in reality they are using MCOs as scapegoats for the loss of benefits and providers and the dwindling accessibility of health care in rural and border communities. MCOs take money away from providers and patients and put it in their pockets calling it "administrative costs". When patients complain to their representatives they take the issue to the state insurance commission. The insurance commission talks to the MCO. A polite letter responds to the representative. The representative calls the constituent and explains how the Governor forced the legislative bill through the legislature. The representative will explain to the constituent how he/she voted against the bill but there were just too many votes against the bill. Legislator assistants will explain that if a bill was passed in support of more accessibility and benefits then the state would have to raise taxes and that most people were against raising taxes.

Monopsony

Large managed care organizations use their market share and financial sheets to gain political health care power. They use their power, size, and fighting skills to bully and overpower others to get what they want. Fee reductions have been one way that these MCOs have used their size to build their bank accounts. This power comes from what is called "monopsony" which is the flip side of monopoly. "In a monopoly, one entity can control all service providers as all mental health professionals. However, in a monopsony one entity controls all of the consumers. Magellan Insurance Company is a managed care organization who is on the way to developing monopsonistic power by controlling the behavior of 40% of the managed mental health consumers in a certain carved out region. This control gives Magellan the power to dictate market terms and fees. Monopsonies as well as monopolies are in clear violation of the Sherman Anti-Trust Act." (21)

Loss of Benefits

Senate Finance Committee Chair Chuck Grassley (R-Iowa) has been quoted as sponsoring a bill to reduce physician reimbursements by 4.3% in Medicare reimbursement that would take effect on January 1, 2006. Senator Grassley said, "What we have is a systemic failure of Medicare payment systems to reward quality." Senator Max Baucus (D-Montana) agrees, adding, "We pay today whether outcomes are good or bad. We ought to pay when outcomes are good." (22)

The Center for Law in the Public Interest filed a class-action lawsuit against the Nebraska Health and Human Services System in June 2004. This suit alleged that Nebraska illegally ended transitional health benefits for single working parents who were no longer eligible for Medicaid because of job changes. "The Transitional Medical Assistance program provides up to one year of coverage for people who have lost Medicaid coverage because they obtained new jobs, received a raise or work new hours that made their incomes higher than the eligibility limits." The lawsuit won Medicaid benefits for about 10,000 single working parents. (23)

There's a new ideological sheriff in charge. Conservative and mainly Republican lawmakers have made the decisions to cut services, make it harder to qualify, and reduce many program in order to keep from raising taxes. "But advocates maintain that what the administration has done is to make a hard road that much steeper. Their biggest complaint is about reductions in child care assistance – the form of help, they argue, that does more than any other to make it possible for welfare recipients to land and stay in jobs." (24) Medicaid has been a safety net for those without insurance and now many are losing that protection. With budget priorities, health and social services have taken a backseat to other programs. Task forces and so-called "blue-ribbon" commissions have been organized and tasked with the job of recommending reform in health care, especially state mental health systems. But the road to hell is paved with unfunded recommendations. Budgetary constraints have left all too many blue-ribbon reports with mildew on the pages. Children with gaps in health insurance coverage commonly do not seek medical care, including preventive visits, and do not get prescriptions filled. These findings are important for both research and policy and point to the need for more encompassing and sensitive measures of the situation of being uninsured. (25)

"An estimated 45 million Americans lack health insurance, and nearly 20 percent of them are children. These kids are often forced to go without medical care, including a pediatrician. 'There are millions of children who are eligible for Medicaid and the State Children's Health Insurance Program, but who are not enrolled. These are uninsured children who are needlessly uninsured,' said Sarah Shuptrine, national program director for the foundation's Covering Kids & Families program." (26)

According to the Urban Institute more than half of the uninsured children in 2002 were eligible for Medicaid and the State Children's Health Insurance Program, but they were not enrolled or lost their enrollment due to lost paperwork. There is the problem with the stigma of big government and the effect this perception has on the population Medicaid is designed to help. Especially in this time of budget cutbacks which directly effect health care providers as well as their patients. "Overcoming these barriers and increasing enrollment often translates into healthier children. And since these government programs cover things such as doctor visits, hospitalizations and prescriptions, they encourage parents to seek primary and preventive care for their children, Shuptrine said." (27)

Shortages of Professionals

Rural America, and especially the border communities, has a significant need for mental health services but there are no or few people willing to drive 150 or more miles to see a few people when the reimbursement rate may not even cover their gas money and lodging expenses. Nevada mental health and development services administrator ranks the inadequate supply of rural clinicians among his top challenges. "Twenty-three percent of the state's mental health jobs in rural areas are vacant. All of my psychiatrists are basically tourists in rural areas." (28)

In Texas there are 52 border counties and each has a shortage of physical and mental health services. In Texas the Texas Drug and Alcohol Commission controls the membership to their organization as well as the funding available. They get most of their funding from

Sustenance Abuse Commission in the Department of Human and Health Services. Over the past few years they were stung by fast-buck specialists and so now they have created a system to slow down the application process for grants and to make application and funding is much more difficult situation for non-profit organizations. Since the agency is not customer-friendly, many agencies that they could and should help either can not afford the application process or choose not to be affiliated with the agency.

Presently there are at least 30 states that are experiencing a shortage of registered nurses and that number is expected to jump to at least 44 by 2020. "The lack of nurses is felt in all sectors: private hospitals, nursing homes and doctor offices as well as facilities run by states and localities – clinics, public hospitals and the like. There is a dearth of nursing teachers to teach the next generation of nurses, thereby cutting down on the number of people who, even if they want to become a nurse, can find an open slot in a nursing program. There are not enough young people being drawn to the profession to replace retiring nurses and meet escalating needs. Lifestyles and demographics are part of the reason. In the early '60s, nursing was one of the few careers open to women. Opportunities are, obviously, greater now, and the supply of students has gone down. Throw state budget problems into the mix and the picture darkens further. Many state schools and community colleges that offer programs to train nurses have been devasated by funding cuts, and early retirement packages to reduce the workforce attracted a healthy share of nursing teachers." (29)

USA Today reported (August 17, 2005) a nationwide shortage of pharmacists in high-growth states such as California, Florida, and North Carolina – and in high rural states such as Missouri, Maine and West Virginia. "The nearly 18,000 independent pharmacies, hospitals, long-term care homes and health insurers also have open positions, while chain drugstores, supermarkets and mass retailers are expected to add 2,200 pharmacies nationwide in the next two years. An increase in prescriptions and aging baby boomers also exacerbate the situation." (30)

Public hospitals are declining in numbers according to a study by the State University of New York's Downstate Medical Center which analyzed data from the nation's 100 largest cities and their suburbs collected by federal agencies. "As a result, there is a major increase in emergency department visits by low-income residents in suburban areas. The study found that low-income patients accounted for about 10.5 million visits to 839 suburban hospitals in 2002. The growth in uninsured people is far quicker than the money available for the public hospitals to care for them." (31)

Failure of Managed Care

Changes in the mental health field over the past 40 years have failed to live up to expectations, creating a fragmented and disorganized system that is scarcely more effective then the one it replaced. When President Kennedy signed the Community Mental Health Centers Act 1963 it signaled the promise of a new regional mental health network, one that would replace the institutional network. Today "millions of people suffering from mental illnesses have struggled – and failed – to maneuver through a web of inadequate emergency, inpatient and community care. What's more, people with private insurance often tap out their mental health benefits quickly and are left to be caught by the public mental health safety net. While there have been some successful government-administered mental health programs, innovation in one county or state is unlikely to be reproduced across the order, particularly in tough budget times. 'The problem with their projects,' says Paul Appelbaum, chair of psychiatry at the University of Massachusetts

Medical School, 'is that they are islands of excellence in a sea of chaos.'" (32)

Some states are bucking the trend. Nevada Governor Kenny Guinn made headlines when he pushed a nearly $900 million tax increase through the legislature, using about $90 million to bolster the Mental Health Department. Nebraska funneled $12 million of its tobacco settlement funds in 2001 and 2002 to expand mental health and substance-abuse programs.

According to the National Coalition managed care "deprives patients of needed treatment, it takes scarce funding away from patients and puts it into administration and profit, it punishes the competent and conscientious professionals, it misleads the public about its effectiveness, and it encourages unethical professional behavior." (33)

The health care movement has failed to live up to the expectations of society. The changes that managed care has brought to health care have failed to live up to all the promises. Instead the health care field is fragmented and disorganized. "Millions of people suffering from mental illnesses have struggled – and failed – to maneuver through a web of inadequate emergency, inpatient and community care." (34) Those that have been stuck in institutions are still stuck. Those who have private insurance are running out of benefits, going bankrupt. "In many cases, states and local governments can't prove their programs work. Contracts with mental health providers tend to emphasize outputs, and outcome measures are few and far between. That means there's little concrete data to prove that money is being spent efficiently and effectively." (35)

Since Medicaid is the safety net for so many people, the amount of money spent on health care is substantial and for mental health along it is estimated by Governing Magazine that Medicaid pays 50% of the national mental health expenditures. Richard Frank, professor of health economics at Harvard Medical School, claims that dynamic between Medicaid and state mental health agencies is a crisis reaching a boiling point. "Now that the state mental health authority isn't the biggest show in town anymore, who has the stewardship for the care of the mentally ill?" (36)

The Costs of Medication Treatment

"Psychotropic drugs, which were introduced with Thorazine in the 1950s, are now the fastest growing line item in state mental health hospital budgets. This is an instance in which the dual goals of quality care and cost control are at odds. There's little question that many of the medications have improved the lives of the mentally ill, and newer drugs have fewer side effects and are more effective than earlier generations. As a result, people are far more willing to continue taking them. The more willing they are to persevere in treatment, the more the cost rises." (37)

Acute care facilities have cut beds as have psychiatric care. With this have come reduced reimbursement rates to providers. As a result physicians and hospitals are opting out of low-reimbursement contracts, such as Medicaid and Medicare. HMOs and MCOs are watching this trend because they have followed the reduced reimbursement rates and fear that the drop-out rate could affect their abilities to maintain quality of services available as well as freedom of choice of primary care physicians which they have advertised. Some states have witnessed psychiatric inpatient beds being turned into more profitable cardiovascular and obstetric beds. Alabama has lost more than 400 psychiatric acute care beds. Without beds patients are left on waiting lists, in ERs, and in jails. Many times patients have to travel more than 100 miles to receive critical care. In 2003 South Carolina had 70 patients waiting for mental health treatment in jail until a state Supreme Court justice ordered the mental health department to find space for them.

One study suggests that half of patients suffering from manic depression, or bipolar disorder, may have been abused as children. Emotional, physical and sexual abuses, or a combination of them, are linked with the condition, which causes dramatic mood swings and changes in behavior. Sexual abuse was also linked to a higher risk of attempted suicide. (38) This study points out how mental illness can escalate over time due to severe childhood trauma. Treatments of such cases normally include medications and psychotherapy.

It's A Jungle Out There!

What ever happened to the paperless society? Trees were supposed to be saved, time saved, lower costs of business but that was just a propaganda ruse. Government agencies and MCOs and HMOs thrive on paperwork because it justifies their existence and because it the public wants accountability and quality. Paper costs money but bureaucrats and employees of MCOs and HMOs don't worry about the costs since they it doesn't come out of their pockets. For the private practitioner, and hospital and the group people are paid to do the job or they have to do it themselves which translates into higher costs of doing business and lower reimbursement rates. Its lower reimbursement rate because there is an increase in demand for additional work without offering additional reimbursements. The computers freeze up in 30 months, the copier runs out of toner and jams up every other week, the fax doesn't want to work, phones are ringing and ringing and ringing…it's a jungle out there.

Now for the issue of "them", those other people who sit-in with us as we do therapy, examining our handwriting, looking at the clock, taking a finger print to insure that the person being seen is who they say they are, though, for all practical reasons, most five-year-olds have a hard time making up a different name for themselves. For my protection, I will change the names of those of who I will discuss. These people have an impact on our practices, on our liability insurance, on our careers, on our financial situation and, for many of these people, on our progress with our patients.

In every state there is one Rooster, one person who functions in the role of governor. Their job is to provide leadership over the legislature, to set priorities, to lead out in the discussion of state problems as well as business development in the state. In case of a catastrophe in the state, this governor is the one who often calls out for peace and calls in the National Guard and phones the federal emergency management agency (FEMA). The Rooster is the one who can say by words or actions, we are not going to raise your taxes and to do that we are going to cut kids and adults off Medicaid or take away their mental health insurance, or make it harder for them to access mental health or dental coverage. We are not going to raise taxes but we are going to raise "sin" habits, car fees, toll road fees, or create toll roads, increase driver license fees, increase gasoline taxes, and maybe another dozen items, but no raise in property taxes or state taxes. The Rooster stands out and waves feathers to direct attention to him/her self and call for people to work harder and sacrifice. He/she will probably say this from their five million dollar mansion or from the yacht that is loaned to him/her. These Roosters are very influential and people in power listen to them, including charity foundations. If the Rooster says we are not going to cut back in mental health benefits, foundations take the clue that they are going to have the same priority. Or/and the Rooster says border-to-border counties are not going to have certain services, that is considered the way of the land.

The next group who has a lot of influence on health care providers is the Lions. The Lions are the leaders of the legislators and they have sergeant-of-arms lions who enforce their opinion and priorities on their fellow legislators. Normally they support the priorities of the Roosters. No lion has ever won a one-on-one political battle in the kingdom of the legislative halls.

The Donkey and Elephant represent the political leadership in each legislative house and their job is to rally their party political legislators to support the "party" policy and priorities. The Dingoes are those who serve as "whips" for their party leadership and their job is to enforce loyalty. The Zebras are the judges who sit on the bench and rule on cases involving health care issues, such as when an individual sues their HMO for refusing authorization for payment for a procedure the patient's doctor says they need. The Hyenas are sent out to attack providers for alleged crimes against the State and humanity, such as over-billing, or failing to document services adequately. Normally they live in the caverns belonging to the State Attorney General. Often joining a hunt are the Buzzards who fly out of the FBI windows to assist in tearing apart offenders. The Wolverines are the Internal Revenue Service representatives who are join the Hyenas in attacking entrepreneurs and health care providers with allegations of "money laundering" or not paying enough taxes. The MCOs and HMOs have their own set of animals such as the pigs that represents the CEOs, CIOs, CFOs, and COOs who conspire to build their fortunes on the backs of providers by cutting reimbursement rates which increases their margins of profit which they then siphon into golden parachutes and bonuses. They also have Tigers auditing the providers' cases looking for ways to cancel their contract for such issues as practicing inefficiently, providing services "not required" and referring too many cases to specialists. Skunks are used to handle pre-authorizations and often complicate the issues by injecting their own scent into the clinical picture and demanding more proof of medical necessity before approving more psychotherapy or a referral for psychological assessment.

Snakes are those who work for the city assessment office and are rather cold and threatening when demanding property taxes. Camels are the bookkeepers, CPAs, and financial advisers that can go on and on and on and not say a thing you can understand and yet their work can get you lost in the desert of tax forms and reports while also protecting you from the legal environmental consequences of not reporting enough revenue or paying enough estimated taxes.

Then there are the Termites from the Board of Examiners who say they are there to protect the citizens of their state, and are the gatekeepers for the license process, but who, in a variety of ways, weaken the whole process of licensing and professionalism by some of their procedures and ways of handling the licensed professionals.

Mosquitoes

No matter what type of organization or group in which we practice our trade, or if we are in a solo practice, we still get the feeling that "they" are out there like a ghost swishing between offices, closets, and even in board rooms. "They" touch our practices, our lives, in more ways then any mystery writer could have prophesied. "They" irritate like pesky mosquitoes, but we fear them as if they were part of the mafia. By definition "they" are people who we never see, we may have never come in contact with them, and they certainly haven't requested any impute from us on any subject of mutual interest. Some times they are politicians, but mostly they are the individuals who write the legislation for the legislators, the bureaucrats, the ones who are the consultants, the "experts", the lobbyists, and the fund raisers. None are medical providers, none are health care providers, and it's probably true that none of them have ever walked in our shoes or felt our collective frustration and pain.

Legislators do not have the background to write bills. Therefore, they hire assistants and specialists who have the background. Those that write legislative bills for health care are normally those who have experience and relationships with corporate America. Many of them may have worked for HMOs and MCOs or legal corporations. These are the worker bees who are said to make honey but in real life sting venom in others causing both pain and despair in health care providers. They write these bills with their personal preferences as a priority. Then the bills are argued in committees and on the floor of the legislature and voted on if it gets that far. The governor and the legislators bicker over whose personal preferences are going to have the highest priority. The decisions to support, or not to support, legislation is determined by who supports the representative or senator. Legislators know what their sponsors want and attempt to please them because they want to keep their job and political position. While most legislators have a legal background others come from business and education fields.

We feel like "they" have stung us despite our efforts to repel their poisonous stings. We are, therefore, the recipients of their unwanted actions. We pay for their success with the loss of our financial success. In fact, they may be basically good family people just doing their jobs. They might not understand how their actions affect our practices. These people (consultants, policy makers, think tank participants, etc.) are operating within the health care marketplace, have a special interest in the hunt, and, in their own companies are pursing wider margins of profit, new business referrals, and ownership of more MCOs and/or medical centers across the nation. This is the business of the health care of which therapy, medicine, surgery, medications are only small slices.

Quality or Quantity

Looking at health care from an economic point of view we have to ask ourselves is do we want to pay for quality or quantity? Some would argue that we need, as a society, is to find a way to pay for how well a service is provided, not on the basis of what's being done.

For example, a 55-year-old male comes in gastrointestinal problems. The doctor offers some medication and makes a follow-up visit. Is the doctor checking for all the possibilities or just treating the symptoms? Should the doctor be paid for each service or how well he is able to solve the patient's problems? One of the quantitative questions might be whither or not the doctor refers this patient to a psychologist for a mental health check-up. Or a middle-aged woman comes in with a history of breast cancer in her family. She complains of nightmares and panic attacks. How well the doctor breaks their symptoms done and refers to other specialists may also be a key to his success in helping their woman over come her fears. Or should we just pay for a mammogram every year?

Currently, the government sits in their ark on the mountain top and collects data about what doctors and social workers and therapists and chiropractors and physical and occupational therapists and psychiatric nurses are doing. They collect data on what treatment is provided for each diagnostic code and their success rate (as measured by the number of sessions seen or procedures provided to eliminate the symptoms). The government pays on the basis of the diagnostic and procedural codes.

It can be argued that we could be spending much more than we are on health care by not paying for some procedures and medications deemed not to have much value. In this vain, we might choose to support preventive medicine programs and care, such as educating parents how to provide better diets for their family, providing more domestic violence prevention education to young adults, offering more support for families with a newborn child, and offering more family support programs for young families in lower social economic communities including high violence areas. In the short term the price of health care would increase but over the long run the costs would be expected to decrease as, we would hope, the costs associated with family violence, postpartum depression, and a decrease in the number of children killed each year by parents or relatives with an anger management or substance abuse problem.

There are two industries in America where we worry about quality: health care and education. In neither do we offer incentives for increased performance value over time.

Power Point

As health care providers we have not done enough to share our opinions and expertise in the marketplace of public opinion. It is time to drop the petty jealousies, protection of "turf" issues, fears of losing "political power" and use our passion for quality health care in support of the common good. It may be our last stand before we are herded into reservations called The National Institute of Health (NIH).

CB&O

End of Chapter Review

Multiple Choice Questions:

1. What are some of the reasons health care providers have shied away from being more active politically?
    a. We don't know how.
    b. We may not know what to say and how to say it.
    c. We may fear that we may become or may be seen as becoming activists.
    d. Lack of trust in the system.
    e. All the above.

2. What do governmental agencies worry most about, in terms of health care, according to this chapter?
    a. Cost
    b. Accessibility
    c. Quality
    d. A, b, and c

3. Policy makers, according to this chapter, are:
    a. Republicans or Democrat legislators
    b. Corporate CEOs
    c. Judges
    d. Political advisors and consultants

4. According to this chapter, politicians do not want to make decisions on:
    a. Eligibility
    b. Accessibility
    c. Entitlement
    d. Costs

5. _____ is fundamental to an entitlement program.
    a. Timing
    b. Accessibility
    c. Funding
    d. Costs

Rethink

1. How has the labor movement lost power and influence in America? And what is the impact on their support of universal health care proposals?
2. Why does large numbers of employed Americans not benefit from employment-based coverage?
3. As a tax paying American, are you entitled to superior health care at any location within your state? Explain.
4. Why hasn't reform efforts succeeded in the past? Or have they? Explain.
5. Discuss the obstacles to people getting the health care that they need.

Personal Observations:

1. Meet with your State Representative and share ideas on health care reform.
2. Meet with your County Judge and share ideas of health care reform in your county. The County Judge is responsible for the MHMR services in your county and could use your input as to how your practice or organization supplement or what services are adjunct to MHMR's.
3. Write a letter to your State Senators expressing your ideas of health care reform.

References

1. Gerston, Larry N., **Public Policy Making**, M. E. Sharpe, NY, 1977, p. 67.
2. Ibid, p. 23.
3. Caller-Times, Scripps Texas, L.P., Corpus Christi, TX, November 5, 2005, p. 5B.
4. Ibid.

5. Walsh, Bill, "Health care bill plays down race", The Times-Picayune, March 30, 2004, www.nola.com/news/t-p/frontpage

6. Office of Disease Prevention and Health Promotion, U. S. Department of Health and Human Services, www.healthypeople.gov/data/midcourse/default.asp

7. Institute for Health Freedom, September 13, 2004, www.forhealthfreedom.org

8. Fact Sheet on the Continued Thickening of Government, www.brookings.edu/printme.

9. Cox/Miami Herald, August 4, 2005, as quoted in kaisernetwork.org

10. Ibid.

11. Hixson, R. R., "Theory L: Management By Leverage", unpublished manuscript, 2006.

12. Stone, Deborah, The Market and the Polis, **Policy Paradox**, W.W. Norton & Company, New York, 2002, p. 21.

13. Huntoon, Lawrence R., The Medicaid Penny, Editorial, Journal of American Physicians and Surgeons, Volume 10, Number 1, Spring 2005, **National Center for Policy Analysis Daily Policy Digest**, January 10, 2005, http://www.ncpa.org.

14. Twila Brase, "How Technocrats are Taking Over the Practice of Medicine: A Wake-Up Call to the American People"

15. British Medical Journal, BMJ Criminal Justice Policy Council, Public Mental Health System in Texas, June 19, 2004, www.cchconline.org/pdfreport/ (Also reported in the Institute for Health Freedom, www.forhealthfreedom.org

16. Governing Magazine, www.governing.com., August 15, 2005

17. Consensus Project, www.consensusproject.org/topics/gp/factsheet

18. Mental Health Association in Texas, Revised 2-28-03, www. mhatexas.org/FACTSHEET1final3_03

19. Surgeon General Finds Mental Disorders Are Common, Drug Benefit Trends 12(1)5-6, 2000, Cliggott Publishing, Division of SCP Communications, www.medscape.com/viewarticle/409888_2

20. Wachino, Victoria, Andy Schneider and David Rousseau, Kaiser Commission on Medicaid and the Uninsured, January 2004, p.4, www.kff.org/medicaid/loadere.cfm

21. Ivan Miller, Ph.D., Potential Monopsony Lawsuit, The National Coalition of Mental Health Professionals and Consumers, www.nomanagedcare.org/lawsuite.html, 6/7/2005

22. www.kaisernetwork.org, July 28, 2005

23. www.kaisernetwork.org, April 8, 2005

24. Greenblatt, Alan, Safety-Net Squeeze, Governing Magazine, June 2005, p. 3.

25. Olson, Lynn M., Suk-fong S. Tang, and Paul W. Newacheck, Children in the United States with Discontinuous Health Insurance Coverage, New England Journal of Medicine, July 28, 2005, pp. 382-391; also read Barbara Starfield, Insurance and the U. S. Health Care System, New England Journal of Medicine, July 28, 2005, p. 418; also read Matthew J. Thibeau and Jeff Tieman, Different Views, Common Ground, The Catholic Health Association of the United States, Health Progress, October 25, Volume 86, Number 5, www.chausa.org/Pub/MainNav/News/HP/Archieve/2005

26. Bhatia, Juhie, Bringing Health Coverage to America's Uninsured Children, HealthDay, August 2, 2005, p. 1, www.healthday.com

27. Ibid.

28. Barrett, Katherine, Richard Greene, Michele Mariani, "Promise Unfulfilled" <u>A Case of Neglect,</u> Governing Magazine, February 2004, p. 6, <u>www.governing.com/archieves/2004/mental</u>

29. Pearlman, Ellen, <u>Brother, Can You Spare An RN?</u>, Governing Magazine, May 2004, p. 1, <u>www.governing.com/archieves/2004/nurses</u>

30. Daily Health Policy Report, January 10, 2005, <u>www.kaiernetwork.org</u>,

31. Ibid.

32. Barrett, et. al., p. 2.

33. National Coalition of Mental Health Professionals and Consumers, <u>www.nomanagedcare.org/Goals&Accomplishments.htm</u>, July 16, 2005

34. Barrett, et al, p. 1.

35. Ibid, p. 2.

36. Barrett, et. al., p. 5.

37. Ibid, p. 4.

38. Garno, Jessica, Joseph F. Goldberg, Paul Michael Ramirez, Barry A. Ritzler, <u>Impact of childhood abuse on the clinical course of bipolar</u> disorder, The British Journal of Psychiatry (2005) 186:121-125, The Royal College of Psychiatrists, <u>www.bjp.rcpsych.org/cgi/content/full/186/2/121</u>

Chapter Five
Financial Whirlpool

Summary

It may not be the first step, but it will be in the top five steps in the development of your private practice. It's as important to your practice as are referrals. Referrals add revenue flow. Financial stability allows you to stay in practice to treat the referrals and collect your reimbursements. While our ancestors depended on their hunting skills to bring food back to the cave, we depend more on our cognitive abilities. This chapter will discuss how financial issues can act like a whirlpool to suck a practice down the drain. Without adequate and timely financial strength we can easily loose what we have worked so hard to develop.

This chapter will help you learn about:

1. Different ways to start your practice and what costs might be expected.
2. Different funding opportunities, or the lack of them.
3. What a profit margin is and how to expand it, and what to do if it shrinks.
4. The "five Cs" of credit
5. How hospitals obtain financing and how ventures play a role in increasing their revenues.
6. The effect of "Deep Pockets" on liabilities and costs of practice.

Square Seven

In this chapter we address the issue of financing, something you may hear a lot about on the state and national arenas. State budgets and the national debt are always being discussed in your state capital and in Washington, D.C. The discussions are the contradictions between what we want and what we can afford. We <u>WANT</u> universal access. We <u>WANT</u> freedom of choice. We <u>WANT</u> to control our costs. The reality is that doing all three, at the same time, may be impossible in today's growing transnational communities in our 50 states.

As a provider you have a dream of helping others resolve their emotional and physical problems and ridding them of diseases and disease so they can return to a state of homeostasis. In every community, having a dream is important. What propels that dream through our illusions and delusions is the cruel reality of a budget and the fact that this month's expenses will be back next month. SBA and bankers will tell you that at least half of new companies will fail before their third anniversary, and one in four will not survive any longer then one year. For those who succeed there are "be" factors that help:

1. Be fully committed to the business project
2. Be driven
3. Be determined
4. Be knowledgeable
5. Be persistent and creative

The first question one normally asks is what is the business you want to startup or purchase? The second question may be, what makes you qualified to run a business? Is your degree from a medical center? Your doctorate may be from the University of Nebraska in Psychology or Social Work, a very good school, but so what? You must like football. Your doctorate in chiropractic medicine is from Parker Chiropractic

School. Good, now go get a license. All these degrees plus your state license give you a background to practice medicine or provide a mental health or social work service, but not one prepares you for what is to come when you open your own practice. Nothing brings this fact home quite like an interview with your banker. "The first step in finding a small business financing is knowing what kind of financing you need. Are you looking for debt financing (money you borrow to run your business) or equity financing (money acquired from investors and/or savings)?" (1)

There are several traditional forms of financing a business: family, credit cards, savings, friends, bank loans, angel investors and private lending. Family and friends can be rather demanding at times if they contribute to your startup capital. They may want weekly reports, and when it takes 15 months to get your first opportunity to start some sort of re-payment plan, they may be very irritable and may even interfere with your business at times. Credit cards are very expensive because they normally have the highest rates of interest. Leasing rather than buying can get you some big items like a car, but at the end of the lease you may regret that you didn't just purchase the items outright. Angel investors tend to be interested in projects over $1 million. Private lenders often consider a project the bank turns down. This brings us back to your meeting with the banker.

Unless you have banked there for a while you will need to provide information about yourself and your business project. Most bankers begin by either meeting you in your office or in the banker's office. Your banker will be a Vice President, but most bankers are Vice Presidents. His or her job is to be your personal banker. Questions of loans are referred to someone else in the bank. Seldom do you have the opportunity to meet with them. This is done because loan requests under $100,000 are handled with a form and an equation. Anything above $100,000 is normally handled by a person with a face, albeit a poker one.

If you don't have a bank account, open one. If you can obtain a credit card, manage it effectively and avoid overdraws, bounced checks and high balances. Borrow a short term-term loan and pay it off within 6 months. Keep your banker informed of upcoming issues like missed projections and payments. Building up a relationship can take some time but can be very rewarding. Over time bankers change banks or are hired by another firm. Therefore, you start all over again with a new banker, but this time there are some credit ratings and bank statements which can improve your chances for a business loan.

Gathering Clouds of Doubt

A good assumption may be that you are reading this because you are interested in entering the health care business, or you are already there and you are looking to find more success. Some of you may feel like you are in the middle of a bridge, and that you are beginning to have some structural deficiencies about which you are harboring some growing doubts. Maybe you expected to have all the answers to your career choice by now. The last time you knew so much and worried so little was when you graduated from high school. Now you have graduated from college with at least masters' degree or even a doctorate. You put so much effort into your grand plan, and you and your family have invested everything you could to reach this point. Your student grants are gone, your scholarships used-up, and your student loan is over six figures! You have six months to find a job before you have to start to pay back the student loan. The clock feels like it's banging each second away in your blood vessels. So let's try to get some perspective.

<u>First,</u> do some basic research; this is called **due diligence**. Contact some mental health professionals in your community and

make appointments to talk about the opportunities in mental health, specifically in private practice or group practice. <u>Secondly</u>, from this information decide (1) if you want to stay in that community, (2) what opportunities might be open to you, and (3) if can you afford to start-up your own practice or should you work with a group practice or a school or hospital. Another option that you may or may not be able to take advantage of at this point is <u>purchasing a practice from someone who is retiring</u> or moving into another direction. <u>Thirdly</u>, take an inventory of your financial health, including your credit history. If you have a bank you have been banking with for over a year, you may choose to approach them about your choices and see how they might <u>view your credit history</u>. They may have some ideas for you since most, but not all, bankers have some experience with health care providers. Some banks are more welcoming to new health care providers, and this interest might serve your needs well.

Bankers' Language

Financing is one of the biggest tasks of your business because of how quickly you can lose everything. If you speak with bankers you need to understand their language. For example, a <u>balance statement</u> is a list of your company's assets, liabilities and equity. Current assets and liabilities are listed separately from long-term assets and liabilities. For your personal <u>financial statement</u> the same list is used. Your financial statements give a clear picture of the company's financial health at any one time. It's easier to manage this by using a software spreadsheet developed by Quicken, Quick Books or Peachtree software. The <u>profit and loss statement</u> is normally a one-year statement but could be longer. This is helpful when comparing one year's profit and losses to another year to find patterns that give you a clue to the success of management. It is also helpful in pinpointing low- and high- performing months.

<u>Performa Notes</u> are statements made in conjunction with the financial statements that explain basic assumptions as well as additional information that could explain expectations or a sudden loss of revenue (e.g., a large number of your patients go on vacation during the summer or are migrants who work up north until October, causing a sudden decline in revenue over four months; or a decline in March might be from school being out for Spring Break; or a decline in certain months may reflect the fact that schools test heavily during these months so that no student can be seen during school hours). <u>Accounts Receivable</u> is a list of billable hours that you have billed for but for which you have not yet been paid. <u>Aging Accounts</u> <u>Receivable</u> indicates how old these invoices or bills are; they tell you when the service was performed and when the insurance company was billed. Accounts are aged to show the period of delinquency (30, 60, 90, or 180+ days delinquent). The longer it takes to collect on a bill, the more of a chance there is of no payment being made.

A <u>business plan</u> is another way to show or tell the banker what you need the money for and what resources you have to pay it back. A business plan might say that you plan to purchase faxes, computers, furniture, and a phone service. The bank can use these for collateral. <u>Cash flow projections</u> are normally done on a spreadsheet with a list of the expected number of patients per week or month multiplied by the amount of money you expect to receive in a certain period of time (45 days, 65 days, etc.). A cash flow projection helps you determine how you are going to meet future expenditures. This type of financial data supports any request for financing. The bank may decide that your business plan is reasonable but that your projections do not allow for a sudden decline in revenue (i.e., you get sick or are in an automobile accident and can't work for several months). The cash flow projection helps the bank assesses the risk of giving you money. <u>Operating income,</u>

or operating profit, is a measurement of the money a company generates from its operations. Operating income can be used to gauge the general health of the business or businesses. The Operating income can be expressed in another way: Operating income = gross profit – operating expenses. If your operating expenses are $60,000 per year and your gross profit is $72,000, then your operating income is $12,000.

A ratio of profitability is calculated as gross earnings divided by revenue, and it measures how much a company makes out of every dollar of services provided. <u>Profit margin</u> is expressed as a percentage; most health care practices are lucky to operate at a 4% profit margin. That statement would mean that for every dollar in sales or services, the company earns four cents. The formula looks something like this: Profit margin = gross profits/total sales or services. The profit margin indicates how much of each revenue dollar your net income is. To understand how this change affects this ratio over time, examine the changes in revenues and expenses.

If you consider the costs of your education an investment, you might be able to use this equation to evaluate, at least financially, the value of your job and income as an investment into your future. If your education cost you $100,000, then your investment is $100,000. If you get $10,000 from family and friends to start up a practice your total investment into your new company is $110,000, plus the time you spend developing the business. After the first year you will want to know what, if anything, you earned on your investment. To find this out you could calculate your annual gross revenue and subtract your total expenses; if there is anything left over, that would be your return on your investments for that year.

<u>Opportunity costs</u> are the result of choices. They are those costs that are of high value at the moment of opportunity, but they result in the loss of an alternative choice once the opportunity is seized. An example

might be the opportunity to rent some space at another office where we can be reasonably assured of a new referral source(s) from one of the other tenants. While we pay rent, payroll and transportation costs at multiple locations, at location One the rent is 55% lower. However, we lose possible new referral sources at location Two. The difference between the two rents minus the estimated difference in revenues in both locations equals the additional revenue we would have lost if we had turned down location Two. Or it shows how much more liable and vulnerable we are in location Two.

A <u>balance sheet</u> is an accounting of all the company's assets, liabilities and net worth. The <u>income statement</u> is an accounting of the total expenses and revenues of the company. <u>Equity funding</u> refers to loans usually secured by the owner's Certificate of Deposit (CD). A CD is paper that says that you have made a deposit of n amount which you agree to leave in the bank for set number of months or years at a certain rate of interest. If you withdraw it sooner you pay a penalty. A CD can be used as collateral on a note.

If you are speaking with a banker you may get some information about the bank's relationship with the Small Business Administration (SBA). The SBA doesn't lend money. Your bank loans money and it needs guarantees and collateral for loans. The SBA offers some guarantee on business loan applications. This guarantee is like collateral on the note. If your business loan application needs additional guarantees or collateral then it can be helpful to work with a bank that understands the value of the SBA and is willing and experienced with working with them. Unless you have a rich family who is willing to give or lend you money or collateral, you will normally need more than good credit to obtain the financing that is going to get you to your fifth year. It's those first few years that push new entrepreneurs off the road to success. Your bank will have a lot of experience working credit cards, car loans and maybe some business loans. Your banker normally takes the application and sends it up to a loan officer who will consider it and then reject it, accept it, or have some questions that might help put the loan together. You may never see this person. If the loan is considered, the application normally returns to your personal bank. Sometimes the banker will know alternative sources for financing as well as for development of a business plan.

Universities normally have a Small Business Development program that assists small businesses in developing business plans in preparation for a presentation with a banker or the SBA. They can offer a variety of programs to help entrepreneurs learn to be more successful. They can also suggest an alternative way of financing your venture, such as a Community Development Loan Fund. These funds are normally supported by local banks and can make certain loans that the regular banking institutions back away from. This Community Fund can accept the note and use funds from the coalition of banks or refer you to an alternative program that offers loans at a higher interest rate.

When you approach a bank for a loan, you will want to come prepared. Knowing the types of questions a banker will ask you will help you be confident and knowledge as you enter what can be a stressful situation. Bankers normally want to know the following:

1. How much money do you need?
2. How are you going to use this money?
3. Will this be a debt loan or equity loan or SBA loan?
4. How much experience do you have in business, this or another?
5. What services will your degree or/and license(s) permit you to bill?
6. What population will be serving?
7. Where are you going to practice?
8. What do you know about the competition in that area?

9. How will you repay this note (loan)?

10. What will you do if you don't obtain this loan?

11. Have you made a business plan?

12. Have you made a three-year projection with Performa notes?

13. Do you have three years of personal tax returns to show your banker?

Banks will provide a copy of an application form and ask for most of the above items. When you make a business plan you will need to list your assumptions which explain why you think you can make money and how you will do it. The Performa notes will explain different parts of the financial statements or spreadsheet, such as the impact of funds or credit or new revenue stream at some point in the three year plan. Most Microsoft computers offer Excell spreadsheets, but there are others. The spreadsheets are good for displaying you estimated expenses and revenues over a period of time.

A business plan normally are about a dozen pages and includes information about the name of the company, its legal status (i.e. non-profit, Sub S Corporation, etc.), the mission and vision statements, organizational chart and information about the management, statements about the market including competition and where your organization will fit (it's niche), information about your product to sell or the type of services and programs offered and what population you will market to and how you plan on marketing your services or products, what environmental or marketplace factors that can be expected to impact positively and negatively on the business throughout the first three years, and a projection of revenues and expenses, what profit percentage is expected and when it is expected (i.e., first year, second year, third year, etc.)

The 5 C's of Business Credit

Bankers with loan authorizations will review you and your company in the context of the 5 C's of small business credit:

- Character - trustworthiness, business experience, knowledge, credit history, references and education.
- Capacity - ability to pay back (available cash flow)
- Collateral - equipment, real estate, inventory, account receivables, securities (CDs, savings, co-signer)
- Conditions - customer base, competitors, liabilities and economics
- Capital - personal capital investment into the company, net worth and equity. (2)

For Start-up Practices

If you are new to the practice of medicine or mental health care, you will want to know what you can expect in a number of ways. This will help you prepare for the worst and accept whatever challenges are facing you so that you can succeed. First, consider your perimeters. What hours can you work? How many hours a week, for how many days? Are you going to take any vacations or holidays off? What are your personal budget needs? If you are in deep debt, maybe private practice is too risky for you now. You may wish to work for an institution such as an insurance company or a hospital or school. If your only debt is a student loan, you may get most of them "forgiven" if you are willing to practice in a rural community. If you are not in serious financial trouble, and have a few dollars saved or have a family and friends who will loan you $30,000, you may wish to consider a private practice. This doesn't mean that you have to rent a building or an office. You may wish to consider sharing space and equipment.

Some office space has a central secretary and receptionist while offering office space with chairs, a couch, a desk and a phone. You can rent this space for a few hours or a day or two per week. This may give you a chance to build up a practice without a heavy outlay of money. It also gives you time to network and develop the need as well as the documentation of the need for your services for future financing applications.

Now comes the time to discuss money, the type that goes out (accounts payable) and the type that comes in (accounts receivable). Your expenses are your payable and when you submit a bill to a HMO or MCO or insurance organization this is your accounts receivable. As you grow these will grow and will need to be monitored by professionals. At that time you may wish to outsource these tasks. When you consider a monthly budget ask yourself: What do I need to live on for the next twelve months? If you need $2500 a month after taxes, and your tax bracket is 33%, then you will need to get paid about $3800 per month. Here is a sample budget:

Rent:	$500 (your rent may include the use of a fax and copier)
Phones:	$250 (with phone call notes)
Supplies:	$150
Professional Dues, Continuing Education Classes, Travel Costs to a Professional Seminar:	$200
Health Insurance:	$360
Payroll:	$2546
Taxes:	$1254
Accounting Fees:	$350
Misc. Expenses:	$200
Total:	**$5410**

To meet this sample budget you will need to see 104 Medicaid patients a month, or 26 per week. I use the lowest reimbursement rate and Medicaid as the provider because you can get paid within two weeks by mail and one week by electronic direct deposit to your bank.

Where can you find 26 patients? Probably not hanging around the mall! If you can get 2 referrals a week it will take you 3 months to reach your goal. To increase this number or to receive a regular flow of patients you will need to be in practice for more than a year unless you have a contract with Child Protective Services or/and a Foster Care Agency. You may choose to work as a contract therapist or psychologist or social worker for another agency until you can build your practice up to 25 to 35 clients per week. It could take a couple of years to reach this goal. When considering your needs, plan on a long-term commitment, not just a 6 to 12 month period of time.

If you rent an office on a part-time basis, can you rent it after 5 p.m. or on Saturdays? If you can afford to quit your day job and start, make sure you have your licenses in place first, and secondly apply for a few panels before you set up your own private practice. A "panel" is the acceptance of the provider by the HMO or MCO to treat patients of the HMO or MCO. The organization then lists your name in their brochure of authorized providers. Normally it can take 2 to 6 months to get on each panel. If you are not on a HMO or MCO panel you are considered "out of network" which means you can not receive reimbursement or you receive a lower amount of reimbursement. **Don't start until you have your license to practice and you have, at the very least, been approved for the following panels: Medicaid, Blue Cross Blue Shield, CHIPS, and a couple of HMOs.** Now, if you have at least six months of income saved up, you are ready to rent some office space. Another option is to rent space with a psychiatrist or a primary care doctor. If you are a medical doctor or chiropractor you may wish to find a practice for sale, or look for contract or part-time work where you see patients in the office one or two days a week for a negotiated price.

For psychologists, social workers, and other mental health therapists, you may wish to connect with some elementary and secondary level schools to see their policy on seeing students at their school. The school counselor normally is the one who is receptive to what your services are and understands the needs at the school. Often it is the counselor who will refer to you. Some schools make a list of providers available to parents to select from for mental health services. Some therapists visit schools, with permission of the parents, and provide play therapy and individual or group therapy in a school room. Sometimes the only room the school has to offer is the school cafeteria. Some school counselors will offer their office. Most schools are appreciative of any help they can get. School counselors are saddled with 300 or more students and a lot of assignments besides counseling students for behavioral problems.

Complacency and Apathy

On-going practices have established policies and procedures, developed a network of referrals, and have had some success financially. At this point an accounting and billing system has been established. Now the management issues beg to be considered so that the agency can progress and not stagnate at a certain level. Not progressing leads to apathy, which leads to lower profits and operational margins, and complacency leads to self-destruction, which adds up to costly mistakes. Referrals decline, paperwork is left for another day, staff and therapists procrastinate, and bills begin to be paid late. Operational costs go up, profit disappear. Dissatisfaction within the ranks increases, as do rumors. People come in late and fail to do follow-ups. The wind of complacency quickly blows dirt into the wheels of progress, slowing or stopping the forward momentum of the practice.

One consultant reported that her clients, a physician partnership, were complaining that they were working harder then ever but their net income was half of what it was the previous year. Some of the problems she discovered that overhead was climbing and collections were down. At the same time, patients complained that they didn't see their doctors long enough to discuss their complaints. The doctors appeared too busy to listen. The consultant also discovered that phones were not being answered from 11:45 a.m. until 2:20 p.m. and some mornings not until 10 a.m. This discouraged patients and referring sources. There's no excuse for that. With an up-to-date fee schedule a physician can make more money without working harder. (3)

Judy Bee, another consultant, concurs that providers need to be more conscious of the business side of business. She was working with one group practice where they were trying to work without an office manager. As a result, the practice was in chaos! The providers claimed they couldn't afford an office manager or administrator. "In that market, an office manager earns about $70,000 a year, and I showed them that they could cover that if each group member generated as little as $11 in additional charges per hour." (3) Practice re-engineering doesn't have to be technical. Changes can be as simple as adjusting your office hours to accommodate your patients. For example, some providers have seen patients at 6:30 a.m. and stopped at 9 a.m. when they made hospital rounds or did networking. Later they returned between 11 a.m. and 1:30 to meet the needs of those who required a lunchtime appointment. Adjusting your hours and your fees to serve a particular patient population, i.e., migrant workers, foster care families, professionals who can only be seen after hours) can add significant income to your balance sheet. Changing your practice hours or marketing to another population are ways to fight complacency, apathy and to rejuvenate your practice.

Health Care Financing

Today hospitals and health care professionals are dealing with issues such as consolidation and collaboration, and each of these issues have financial and legality implications. While some hospitals have merged, they face legal action by federal and state agencies that can accuse them of monopolizing services in a marketplace. The primary purpose of consolidation and collaboration efforts (through mergers, affiliations, systems, partnerships) is to create more leverage with insurance companies, including managed care companies. These efforts arose because managed care was offering contracts that did not let physicians and other health care providers negotiate a contract. Physicians had to either accept a proposed contract or not be able to see patients from that managed care health network without making the patient pay large deductible plus higher co-payments. Health care providers have resented the intrusion of insurance bureaucrats into the doctor-patient or therapist-patient relationship. Therefore, other legal entities have been formed in order try to the increase the reimbursements and decrease the amount of intrusion.

Independent practice (provider) associations (IPAs) were formed in the late 1980s and early 1990s. By definition, IPAs represent only physician interests. Managed care companies would first negotiate with hospitals and later with IPAs. For the most part, managed care companies didn't care who got the "better" contract. But it has meant a great deal to IPAs, who have often fought for conflicting contracts with managed care companies. To reduce this conflict, physician-hospital organizations (PHOs) were formed as a joint venture or partnership. In these relationships the physicians and hospitals share in the ownership and governance of the PHOs. Another legal structure created to administer primary care practices were hospital-affiliated group practices (HAGPs) which often taken one of two forms. One form has the hospital directly employing the primary car physicians, while in the second form a specialized corporate subsidiary becomes the employer. "A few hospitals have created management service organization (MSO) subsidiaries that acquire the business assets of a medical practice and employ all the administrative personnel needed to perform claims processing, billing, patient scheduling, and other important management functions." (4)

Hospitals receive funding in a number of ways. Among these are grants, charitable contributions, sliding scale fees (based on ability to pay), straight charges, and some form of discounts. In addition to these provides the following model for reimbursing hospitals:

- Per diems (negotiated per day rates for an HMO, insurance company, state or federal agency).
- Differential by each day a patients spends in a hospital (usually the first day rate is higher due to additional services).
- DRG (diagnosis-related groups).
- Differential by service type (negotiated by service such as medical, surgical intensive care, neo-natal intensive care, psychiatry, obstetrics, etc.).
- Case rates or package type (negotiated rate for categories of procedures such as obstetrics).
- Capitation or percent of revenue
- Penalties and withholds (negotiated goals for length of stay, if met or exceeded, then the hospital receives its withheld funds or a bonus, if not met, they are not paid the withheld funds or bonus).
- Outpatient care (negotiated discounts, flat charges, case rates or capitation). (5)

Psychiatric hospitals and outpatient medical clinics are among these hospitals included in one or more of the above charges. Outpatient mental health services normally fellow the discounted, sliding scale, contracts or grants and charitable contributions. Contracts are negotiated between an organization and a mental health organization to provide mental health services to certain identified populations.

Cost Control Mechanisms' Effect

Managed care organizations were created to control costs, but they are failing in many ways. ""Reasonable price" as well as "quality care" are being debated in different think-tank circles as well as by those who are responsible for health care financing, including MCOs. Physicians and other professional health care providers desire more interdependence in health care delivery and less dependency on bureaucratic administrators. Patients want unlimited access and freedom of choice. The government wants more appreciation for and less criticism of their Medicaid and Medicare programs. MCOs want to maximize profits. Health care providers also want to control costs and show a profit. This creates a basic contradiction in the debate over financing health care. "Choices for change must recognize these contradictions in a way that enables all the key players to participate in a cooperative strategy to reform the system. That means they're going to have to think about the fundamental values that have driven their behavior up to this point." (6)

"We have moved from small businesses to large businesses within the health care field, from a pattern of individual practice to group practices in hospitals and elsewhere. We have moved from community hospitals rooted in a particular place and tradition to the development of very large chains. We had a recent merger that will give us a chain of something like 140 hospitals. This size and complexity puts pressure on our efforts to recognize traditional values and make them effective." (7)

While primary care physicians have been the primary gatekeepers to health care services, many others have been added, such as chiropractors and internists, who have become the "treating physician" in many cases (workers' compensation, etc.). A gatekeeper for an HMO is the primary care physician. Recent changes in managed care forces patients to receive a referral to a specialist, often from the gatekeeper who is the Primary "care physician (PCP). And sometimes the HMO or MCO will have a list of specialists they will authorize services. Often this requires time and consultation with the HMO pre-authorization department. During the 1990s, and even today, HMOs pay primary care physicians cash for their practices and offer them employment contracts varying from 3 to 5 years. Many of them just receive salary or income guaranties like $6 a month for 3000 to 4000 patients. They receive this income whether they see the patients or not. Thus the HMOs are influencing and hopefully, by their point of view, controlling primary care physicians who feel obligated to hesitate before referring patients to specialists.

By definition "managed health care, or managed care, is an approach to managing both the quality and the cost of medical care.... In general, there are at least two elements common to managed health care systems: an authorization system and some level of restriction imposed on a member's choice of providers. The authorization system may be minimal, such as a simple hospital precertification requirement; or it may be comprehensive, such as a primary care physician (PCP) gatekeeper model. The restriction on choice of provider can be minimal, such as minor increase in co-insurance to see an out-of-network provider in a preferred provider organization (PPO); or it may be strict, such as in a highly restrictive health maintenance organization (HMO)." (8)

Managed care can be viewed as a continuum of models ranging from:

a. Indemnity with precertification (protecting against loss by requiring precertification), mandatory second opinion, and large case management;

b. Preferred Provider Organizations (PPOs),

c. Point of service (POS),

d. "Open access" HMOs,

e. Closed panel HMOs.

As these models change, so does the control of the service and patient:

a. Elements of control over health care delivery become tighter,

b. New elements of control are added,

c. Greater control of utilization is made, and

d. Net reduction in rate of rise of medical costs occurs. (9)

One of the deterrents to seeing patients has been "open" and "closed panels." Open panels are insurance companies that accept new providers. In an open panel any willing provider which means any independent contractor that is willing to accept the insurance organization's conditions and standards. Closed panels do not accept new providers. A "closed" panel system is one where the total number of physicians or providers is much less than in any other model. Usually the HMO pays a group a negotiated capitation, and the group pays the providers through a combination of salary and risk/reward incentives. The group is responsible for its governance and partners. Usually the HMO is responsible for the practice facility and the support staff. The group shares in the risk of the practice in that if the group exceeds the capitation amount, the HMO lowers the reimbursement to the providers, although there is generally a stop-loss insurance coverage to the group to protect the group from catastrophic cost overruns.

More and more providers of Medicaid are dropping out of the program for several reasons:

1. Medicaid patients have the highest no-show rates

2. Medicaid patients tend to demand the most time and attention

3. Medicaid pays the lowest rate

4. Medicaid MCO administrators change so often that it is confusing and costly to providers.

5. Medicaid MCO administrators, to include the administrators of the traditional Medicaid program, are not provider-friendly. It is very hard to get a "straight" answer, at least the same answer, from different sources within the provider-relations department.

6. The liabilities are higher, and there is a slim to no profit margin. Providers have to constantly fill out paper work such as new credentialing forms, new provider forms, and extension of services forms.

7. It takes six months or longer to get a new therapist on a company provider list; Medicaid administrators have found another way to delay access and to hurt providers, not to mention the patients who have to either find another provider who will take them or go to the emergency room.

8. The only option to no-shows is to "fire" oneself from treating patients who abuse one's practice. In metropolitan areas the patients have more options, but in rural communities a provider is often the only one there. This translates into seeing the patient having to see his or her PCP or traveling 150 miles to a metropolitan area provider. The PCP may be happy to

charge for an office visit, but the PCP is not a mental health provider.

Legislators are faced with critical questions and decisions. They are provided with information from lobbyists, think tanks, consultants and a host of organizations that provide information such as Kaiser Family Foundation and publications such as *Health Care Management*. There are myths that affect the cost-effectiveness of health care and the bottom line for health care providers. One such myth states that the more children are enrolled in Medicaid, the higher the costs of health care for the states. In reality children are the cheapest group to cover, and prevention in this age group pays off. "Children and their parents make up 73 percent of the Medicaid covered population but only 25 percent of the health care spending." (10)

According to Ku and Guyer, very little of the growth of Medicaid spending is due to children, because per capita costs are quite low. In FY 2000, $200 million in increased federal Medicaid spending was due to adding children and adults, while. $1.8 billion in increased spending was due to state fiscal strategies. (11)

The Impact of Having Deep Pockets

As you begin to add all this information together, hopefully you can see how we are in the middle of a triangular tug-of-war with governmental agencies, HMOs and the general population all pulling us at the same time in different directions, attempting to control us, to use us, to manipulate us, to blame us and then to showcase us as the best in the world. Practicing defensibly is critical to survival, but cannot guarantee survival.

We have discussed primarily private and group practice vs. hospitals to show the clear difference in billing codes and procedures and how large groups (PPOs, multi-specialty groups) and HMOs, MCOs, etc.

have more financial flexibility and deeper pockets of funding and insurance. **Large practices and organizations have the resources to handle frequent changes; private practitioners do not have these resources.** Large organizations buy specialists to handle tasks that help defend their group practice or their administrative roles and funding sources. They outsource human resource departments, retain teams of lawyers, purchase the services of compliance teams, retain cost-effectiveness programmers and teams, utilize computer experts and hire nurses to call those cases that are likely to be long-term drains on their financial resources. HMOs and workers' compensation insurance organizations enjoy the luxury of having case managers who go further looking for ways to terminate treatment reimbursements. It makes sense for the HMOs but may interfere with the provider's efforts and plan of action to help people get well and learn better coping mechanisms so they can return to work or to a more functional position in the family and community again.

Private practitioners do not collect enough revenue to hire all these people and pay for all these services. Therefore, we are at the mercy of the wind and the whims of bully insurance organizations. Having "no pockets" can be helpful at times because most attorneys will not consider taking action against such agencies as worthy of their time and effort. Most professional liability policies will be around a million dollars for physicians and maybe as low as $300,000 for therapists. That is why group practices carry so much insurance and have teams of attorneys on retainer. Hospitals are the same. They are much more likely to be hit with a monster lawsuit then those in private practice. However, such lawsuits can happen to private practices, and when they do happen there may be other names on the indictment. It isn't just that one may be sued, but if you are sued, even when you win the case, you are likely to lose your practice because of the cost of defining yourself, including defining yourself to your referral sources and professional associates. Then, of course, there are the emotional costs. There are things we can do, a way to fight back; a way to survive audits, lawsuits, allegations of fraud and the second half of this book will discuss them.

Power Point

Since this is a business we need to be more aware of how to operate within the health care marketplace and we need to know how to talk "business" or "banker's" talk. It's important to be able to understand our patients in English, Spanish, Koran, etc. So it is necessary to know the language of our CPAs and Bankers.

End of Chapter Review

Multiple Choice Questions:

1. According to this chapter, which of these is MOST likely to get a loan? While all of them may get a loan, the one you choose is the one that has the best chance, with everything else being equal.
    a. A surgeon who is billing over a million a year.
    b. A primary care physician who is billing over 300,000 per year.
    c. A chiropractor or physical therapist who is billing over $150,000 a year
    d. A marriage and family therapist who is billing over $70,000 a year.

2. There are several traditional forms of financing a business. Two of these include:
    a. Credit cards and family
    b. Angel Investors and Banks
    c. Savings and Angel Investors
    d. Factoring and friends

3. Accounts Receivable is
    a. A list of your revenues
    b. A list of your creditors
    c. A list of billable hours that you have sent out
    d. A list of assets, liabilities and equity of your company

4. Cash flow projections is
    a. A way to show your banker what you need money for
    b. A measurement of the money a company generated from its own operations
    c. A list of invoices that has been aged by 30 and 60 day periods of time
    d. A spreadsheet with a list of expected number of patients per week or month multiplied by the amount of money you expect to receive in a period of time.

5. The 5 C's of Business Credit includes:
    a. Character, Capacity, Conditions, Capital, and Currency

    b. Character, Capacity, Currency, Capital and Credit Amount

    c. Character, Currency, Credit Amount, Collateral, Conditions

    d. Conditions, Capacity, Capital, Collateral, and Character

6. The summer of 1982 saw the adoption of legislation that effectively ended _____ reimbursement to hospitals for Medicare patients and replaced it with prospective payment, based on diagnosis-related groups.

    a. Fee-or-service

    b. Cost-based

    c. The Workshop Model of

    d. Projective costs

7. Opportunity costs are those costs that are:

    a. Of high value at the moment of opportunity

    b. An alternative choice later

    c. Highest cost

    d. Of low value at the moment of opportunity

8. Not _____ leads to apathy, which leads to lower profits and costly mistakes.

    a. Networking

    b. Marketing

    c. Managing

    d. Progressing

9. According to this chapter the earliest hospitals were created for those who got sick and:

    a. Had money and prestige

    b. Had position in the community

    c. Had no home

    d. Orphans and widows

10. A gatekeeper for an HMO is typically a:

    a. Psychologist

    b. Psychiatrist

    c. Chiropractor

    d. Primary Care Physician

ReThink:

1. Explain some of the reasons that businesses fail in their first three years.

2. Explain what "due diligence" means and how it is performed.

3. Develop a likely monthly budget for the first twelve months, putting in notes below each month of anticipated billable hours and how summer vacation or Spring Break or holidays might influence your revenue flow.

4. Compare monthly revenues and expenses between a possible private practice and joining a group either as a full-time employee or a part-time contract worker. Balance the advantages and disadvantage of each practice for you at this time in your life and practice.

Personal Observation:

Contact the nearest Small Business Development program and make an appointment with a counselor and review services they provide and how it might help you get started in your private practice. Secondly, gather information about lease and rental property that might be attractive to you.

References

1. Ward, Susan, Finding Small Business Financing, About.com, June 14, 2005, p. 1, www.about.com/cs/bestpractices.

2. Zahorsky, Darrell, New Rules of Small Business Financing, About.com, June 14, 2005, pp. 1-2, www.about.com/cs/bestpractices

3. Weiss, Gail G., Big Practice Problems, Medical Economics, Dec. 17, 2004, p. 2, www.memag.com/memag/article

4. Ibid.

5. Rosenfield, Robert H., The Legal Structure of Health Care,

Health Care Administration, 3rd Ed., Lawrence F. Wolper, ED., Aspen Publication, Maryland, 1999, pp. 89-90.

6. Ibid, p. 93.

7. Kongstvdt, Peter R., Managed Health Care, **Health Care Administration**, 3rd Ed., Lawrence F. Wolper, ED., Aspen Publication, Maryland, 1999, p. 530.

8. Bernard R. Tresnowki, "The Necessary Debate: Resolving Contradictions", Health Care Ethics: Business Aspects, **Woodstock Report**, December, 1993, #36, p. 4, www8. georgetown.edu/centers/woodstock/publications/report/r-fea36.htm.

9. Langan, John P., "Balancing Values and Adjusting to Change", p. 5, Ibid.

10. Kongstvedt, Peter R., Managed Health Care, **Health Care Administration**, 3rd Ed., Lawrence F. Wolper, ED., Aspen Publication, Maryland, 1999, p. 523.

13. Ibid, p. 524

14. Ladenheim, Kala, Carrie Farmer, Donna Folkemer, Wendy Fox-Grage, Kevin Horahan, Anna Scanlon, Tara Shaw, Managing Medicaid Costs: A Legislator's Tool Kit, National Conference of State Legislatures, March 2002, www.ncsl.org/programs/health/forum/cost/containment.htm

15. Ku, Leighton, and Jocelyn Guyer, "Medicaid Spending: Rising Again, but not to Crisis Levels, Washington, D. C.: Center for Budget & Policy Priorities, 2001, www.cbpp.org/4-20-01health.htm, as quoted in Managing Medicaid Costs: A Legislator's Tool Kit, National Conference of State Legislatures, March 2002, www.ncsl.org/programs/health/forum/cost/containment.htm

Part Two

Techniques and Tools For Finding and Dismantling
Road Mines to Successful Practice of Health Care

Chapter Six
Looking For a Rock Foundation

Summary

This chapter discusses the development of a strategy to start-up a practice; join a group practice or purchases an on-going practice (private or group). Other options are also discussed, such as joining a multi-specialty practice, non-profit organization or hospital psychiatric ward or accepting a school counseling position. Additionally, you will learn about choosing a location for the practice and determining the type of population and economic background you will serve. You will also read about developing a sales and business plan while you create a practice vision and mission statement. These plans and statements effect how and where you practice. These issues are important as you develop a practice that can withstand the storms of winter including hurricane floods.

After reading this chapter you should be able to do the following::

1. Discuss the different types of practices that may be available to you.

2. Determine which type of practice might be a priority at this point in your life and career.

3. Discuss the advantages and disadvantages of practicing in urban, suburban and rural communities.

4. Discuss the effects of economic factors that may affect access to adequate health care.

5. Discuss how cultural diversity and traditions may effect the

growth or demise of a practice.

6. Write a vision and mission statement.

7. Explain the value of a business plan in a start-up practice.

Off-Ramp to the Sharp and the Jagged

This is your life, your practice. It defines who and what you are. You have spent years in school and in preparation for this time. The costs of an education are high. And it is unbelievably cheap. Asking a college or university to do in four to eight or nine years when your parents couldn't do in 18 years is quite a request. Many professors, including adjunct professors, are glad you arrived for classes. Maybe "glad" is too vibrant a word. Perhaps satisfied is better. When I attended the first years of college, they were glad I had shoes on (dirty and holey tennis shoes).

After all the undergraduate and graduate course work and celebrations for surviving, you may be facing a new uncertainty: unadulterated confusion. Most must spend another two years paying for the right to take the state licensing examination! The upside is that you now can get a paycheck, albeit a small one and you have the time to research how you want to use your expensive education. Many people think that once they have gotten through all this they have completed the worst part of their educational lives. Welcome to Life 101! The next phase of your education has just begun.

Private Practice

Private practices are drying up and their practitioners have been embracing group practices. They are casualties of managed care, having faced the extreme hardship of having to practice in a hostile climate. It can be too much for anyone to effectively and efficiently do it alone. After reading the previous chapters you might conclude that you want to find a niche with a multi-specialty group or a group of behavioral health or primary care providers to lower costs, and to decrease the lone wolf or ranger syndrome.

It takes time to develop a strategy for developing your own practice, buy into an established group practice, or become a contract employee or a contract self-employed person. Private practice doesn't mean you have to have an office in a building away from other practices. You may find a group that shares office space or/and secretarial support services with other therapists or professionals. You still have to do your own billing and install your own computer, phone and fax lines. You may be able to share computer expenses. You can handle your bank account balancing, especially if you have an accountant or CPA handling the tax returns. You may have no fringe benefits the first few years. Vacations are a luxury.

Location, Space, Telephone Service

Location is an important decision and sets the tone for type of services you will offer as well as populations you may want to see. If you locate an office in a low social economic community, a majority of your cases will be funded by Medicaid. If you do not speak another language besides English, or if you prefer to handle more HMOs business then Medicaid, you will have to find an office in a location where you can see these populations. When you can afford a receptionist you may want to select one who can speak one of the other languages of the community.

Location needs to be accessible to public transportation and have adequate parking spaces. You could need a private office, a reception area, a billing and collection room or space, perhaps a second office for another therapist or physician, and a room to do play therapy, if you plan on seeing a lot of children, or a room to do training in, such as parenting class to several parents. Other space you may want is a kitchen area and a storage room plus a private restroom. Your building needs to have a restroom for males and one for females on each floor and if they are locked you will need a key. Put that key on something larger than a pocket or that is hard to get into a purse. You can do with less, but at some point you may want to expand or invite another professional to share offices and sharing office expenses. If you don't want to break a lease, and there isn't enough space in your building, knocking out walls may want to be considered. Also, seeing patients across the city or in another town or sharing office space with a group practice are all options to think about. <u>Keeping expenses down will be one of your most important jobs during your first five years</u>.

Telephone service can be one phone and SBC Call Notes that saves your messages. Or you can have the phone transfer to your cell phone. Or, if you sharing space with a receptionist, the receptionist can answer your calls. Purchase a cell phone so you can stay in touch with your office even when you are out of the office. Purchasing a multiple local phone connections can cost $3,000 plus to purchase and install.

Selecting office space means giving thought to easy access for patients. Office space should be compliant with the American's with Disabilities Act and have space available for wheelchairs. There should also be sufficient space for parking, as your patient load will usually rely on their vehicles rather than depending on public transportation or a ride from a relative.

Practicing by yourself can feel very lonely, especially if you practice in rural communities. There is an increase in self-pitying thoughts and behaviors; this is often referred to as "burnout". In order to avoid burnout you can give yourself a few years working with an organization, learning the ropes and taking time to develop your own reputation, which will translate into more referral sources once you leave the agency. It will also give you a support network of other professionals who can help you later on down the road. Find a mentor and let that person bill for you, refer to you, and take a reasonable percentage of collections to reimburse his/her expenses. This will also help you to learn the intricacies of diagnosis. Learning to listen and make effective treatment plans is very important. Real life symptoms are not perfect matches for each case. In addition, patients are not always accurate historians of their mental, physical and medical experiences. When you ask them about the mental health problems of their family, or those of their spouse, they don't always know, and secondly, they may have been told that Mom had a nervous breakdown but not that she became so depressed that she because suicidal.

You might consider working out of your home. Also, you can see patients by going to the homes of patients or seeing them in the front room or office in your house or apartment. Of course, there are drawbacks to this type of practice. Whenever you practice in your home or apartment you invite liabilities that you might not get when seeing patients in an office. Men and women can be accused of making unwanted advances to patients. It may not be true, but the cost of defending yourself will be expensive.

Going to homes can bring the liabilities above, but when you visit the homes of patients you also face the potential for physical violence against you. I have had the experience of being in a home when drive-by shooting occurred down the street. Another time I was in a home when a drunken man came to the home saying he wanted to explain what he did earlier in the day. The family I was with had reported to me that this man had pushed down their six year old by and said some ugly things. The boy's father was very upset, and when he heard this man outside his house talking to the boy's aunt and grandmother, the boy's father went for his gun. The boy's mother went outside to get the man to leave, and I was left there trying to stop an angry father.

It was a very tough situation. Fortunately this wasn't the first time I had seen the family. They trusted me, and so the father stayed in the house until his wife returned to tell him the man had apologized and left. The drunken guy was stupid but not dumb. The boy's father was known in the community to deal out his own type of justice. The man probably saved his own life in apologizing and in agreeing never to talk to or touch the boy and his family again.

Other times I have been in the home when someone bursts into the house and accuses the man or woman of infidelity. Having a cell phone can be a good way to call for police assistance. Other times I have arrived at the home to find some one who has overdosed, or who has refused medication and is threatening to jump out of the 4th floor window. Another time the lady of the house was a heroin addict and "coming down" and was very agitated. Another time a neighbor thought I was there to take the kids away and set two Pit bulls on me. Many neighborhoods people know what the problems are but try to "protect" their neighbor who they know against outside agencies like Child Protective Services and the Police. Working in homes or being on-call can bring any number of dangerous situations.

Legal Entities

The legal structure of a practice needs to be considered due to both legal and financial liabilities. Sole practitioners operate without being incorporated. **Sole proprietorship** means that you operate your business under your name and that you are the only owner of the company. Some file notarized "dba" (doing business as) papers with the city clerk. Others form a state corporation under their name or a fictitious name and then file appropriate dba forms with the city clerk. State corporations can be **"sub-S" corporations** (S corporations), which have distinct tax benefits for the owner. Corporations for general business (as opposed to those formed for a specific purpose, as stated on their corporate paperwork with the state) are often referred to as **"C corporations"**. These have fewer limitations then S Corporations but come with a double taxation for the owners because the corporation gets taxed once and then the owners get taxed on their share. The S Corporation limits the number of shareholders, limits the amount of business losses that can be passed on to the shareholders and limits some fringe benefits that can be passed on to the owners as business expenses. Always consult your attorney and CPA when discussing issues that effect liabilities and finance. The attorney will ensure you complete the right paperwork and the CPA will keep your fingers off of the IRS's stove. Another type of corporation is the **limited liability corporation (LLC),** which is organized and operated for a limited purpose. Then there is the professional corporation or professional association (PC) (PA) that often applies to defined groups of professionals such as medical doctors and attorneys. You can form a corporation with partners and each one of you will be issued "x" number of shares. You will have a Board of Directors and/or a General Manager or Managing Partner who will act as the official spokesperson for the organization and will sign any official papers.

According to Budman and Steenbarger, a corporation has four characteristics:

- Limited liability. Owners of a corporation are shielded from tort and contract claims arising against the firm. Torts are civil action as opposed to criminal actions. Legal actions include law suits of injuries caused by your practice.
- Continuity of existence. The existence of the corporation does not depend on its ownership. Changes in ownership do not necessitate the dissolution of the firm.
- Transferability of ownership. Ownership in the corporation is

facilitated by the issuance of shares of stock to owners. These shares are easily transferred from one party to another in the event of an owner's retirement, death, bankruptcy, and so on.

• Centralized management. Corporations have a designated board of directors empowered to run the firm. (the Essential Guide to Group Practice in Mental Health, Guilford Press, New York, 1997, pp.94-95)

Group or Multi-Specialist Practices

Working as an independent practice within an office of other specialists and primary care physicians can be very helpful. You share expenses, get some referrals, and are close enough to learn from more experienced therapists or physicians. If you can afford the start-up costs and can get through 3 to 5 years practicing like this you could do well, but there is no guarantee. However, it can be a very good learning experience. Working with other professionals can provide unlimited expertise to your practice and increase your effectiveness with you patients.

Working for an organization can be a way to start your practice. The advantage is that you start out with a caseload. Secondly, the organization may be willing to do all the billing and collections and give you a salary. A third advantage is that you have an office, phones, answering service, and secretarial support. A fourth advantage is that the organization will have an attorney that represents the corporation, and they get legal assistance from which you might benefit. A fifth advantage is that they already have name recognition. A sixth advantage is that they usually have regular staffing or/and training that you couldn't afford by yourself. A disadvantage is that you have to bill "x" number of hours per week to keep your salary. A second disadvantage is that you will be expected to help them develop additional referral sources. A third disadvantage is that you work for someone else.

Practice Collaboration

Practice collaboration doesn't necessarily mean that individual practitioners join group practices, though that could happen. Practice collaboration also means more than just a few consultations between the primary care doctor and the psychologist or chiropractor. "For years, the health care professions – including the mental health fields – were largely solo enterprises. This is rapidly changing, as practitioners recognize the benefits of affiliation. By linking to other professionals, they can create convenience for customers and professional and financial synergies for themselves. These are clusters of solo private practices yoked to psychiatric practices (also solo) for the purposes of case consultation, cross-referral, marketing, and contracting. Participants in the Professional Affiliation Groups (APG) can offer a wide array of services to clients and referral sources, generating increased business. They also enhanced professional communications and innovative mechanisms for case management and cost control." (Budman and Steenbarger, 1994, p. 5)

Although such collaboration still exists today, they are not nearly as prevalent or strong as they were ten years ago. There are several reasons for this, including the following:

1. Collaboration success is built when practitioners share time, expertise, and resources. When physicians, therapists and social workers feel that they are referring more then is referred back to them, or that information they provide is more one sided, they begin to hold back. This weakens efforts to develop a working collaboration network.

2. New laws that attack any "scheme" or "strategy" for "payment"

for referrals have hampered efforts to generate referrals by paying for office space or consultant fees, etc.

3. MCOs and HMOs are developing a system for controlling for costs re-defining the gatekeeper position. Assigning primary care physicians (PCPs) the job of completing more forms to request a referral to a specialist for additional tests can act as a way to discourage any referral to a specialist (mental health, physical therapy, neurological assessments, etc.)

4. New federal regulations (HIPPA and Sarbanes Oxley) have discouraged some exchanges and puts emphasize on accurate accounting systems. While the Sarbanes Oxley Act has more of an effect on hospitals and larger groups it issues a warning to others not to "cook the books" (financials and tax returns).

5. Current collaborations are fairly loose in organizations with few strong leaders. At times some educational organizations attempt to be the leader but often are not very effective since they are viewed as "not one of us". This means that they may encourage other professionals to call them for advice and possibly using them for consultations, or using their graduate school counseling centers as a resource. Many graduate school professors are writing a book or doing research and ask for referrals for these purposes more than adding something to the local community clinicians. Collaboration only works when those collaborating take responsibility to refer within the group of collaborators.

Multispecialty and collaboration groups continue in theory and practice, but they remain the exception to smaller groups and individual practices. Still, changes in the marketplace spur innovation and the discussion of ways to react to increasing pressures by both the government (priorities in budgets, additional regulations and increased aggressive prosecution), more administrative fees from MCOs, lower reimbursement rates for providers and more "filters" and infringements on practice management all in the name of "quality assurance" and "cost effectiveness." Such vice-like pressure on health care professionals of all disciplines discourages those who invest in private or small group practices and jeopardizes the quantity and quality of care, despite the United States "having the best health care in the world." It is rather ironic that those who make these claims on television and in the print media are many of the same individuals who are leading the way to bring down individual and small group health care providers and forcing some type of governmental takeover. In this atmosphere the community of health care providers needs creative approaches and new ways to thinking of costs and what we get in return for those costs. Although we may already vote, that is no longer enough.

Working for a Non-Profit Community Service Organization

Non-profit organizations are formed by contributions from individuals who apply some of their earnings back into the company to pay for the legal and financial creation of the agency. Non profits are often financed by grants, insurance reimbursements, and contributions from local organizations.

Working for these organizations usually means having an instant caseload, doing extra paper work, and being part of a team. Usually salaries are in the low to medium range for the geographical location. Salaries and operating expenses are funded with grant money, individual contributions and insurance reimbursements. This means if a grant ends, there will be downsizing within the organization. Working for a non-profit organization that may lose all or part of its grant funding each year can be quite jarring for some. Well established community service organizations are not usually at the mercy of business trends or changes in state budget priorities; smaller and newer for-profits tend to be more at the mercy of these forces because they lack the established infrastructure and broader funding base of the larger and older nonprofits.

Working for a Hospital's Psychiatric Ward

Working for an acute care hospital with a psychiatric and/or substance abuse ward has become popular again. Ten years ago these wards were shutting down under the cloud of suspicion of insurance fraud. Some psychiatric hospital chains such as the Brown Schools continue. Others have sold out or have closed down. HCA hospital chain remains open but under a drastically different setting then ten years ago.

At one time substance abuse programs offered 30-day inpatient care. Now they have a hard time getting approval for a 3-day detoxification program. There are some specialty hospitals that can provide longer-term care for teenagers with frequent drug abuse problems. For longer-term mental health problems there are fewer programs. State hospitals have longer-term programs, primarily for adults with some for adolescents. With budget cutbacks beds are being lost and positions cut.

Working as a School Counselor

Some graduate students complete their master's work in counseling and go on to finish the requirements for a license. Then they stay in school and work as school counselors. Some complete requirements to allow them to obtain a principal's position and then advance to a position with more responsibilities, such as a Superintendent position. Few ever work in private practice. There may be good reasons for this, including the issues of security. Educational institutions can provide a very sound and secure job and a very good retirement. Most educators have many more days off then do other professions, especially when compared to the mental health field. There are, however, therapists and psychologists who have reached a point where they can take one day off each week, for leisure activities or writing, but it often takes them quite a few years to get to this point.

Location of a Practice

Urban – The Office of Management and Budget defines metropolitan areas as those with 50,000 or more inhabitants. (Miller, 2002, p. 1) Working in a metropolitan area like this can be very challenging. It's not always cheap, nor is there much space. Finding a group practice, or find a group who shares office space and expenses but are independent of each other, can be rewarding. Normally a new member is accepted into the group if he or she specializes in a treatment or diagnosis that the others do not, or where there is an abundance of cases and a lack of people willing to work with a given population (e.g., adolescents with a conduct disorder, oadults with borderline personality disorder or children with ADHD). A disadvantage of working in an urban area is that there could be a large Medicaid population. .

If you work in a metropolitan community you may drive 15 or 30 minutes to work during heavy traffic times, and you don't have to pay for a hotel room and eat out. When you travel you carry your files. If you do play therapy, you carry a bag of toys, perhaps with several games. Whenever you move things from one location to another you have the chance of losing them: paper work, toys, games, important information.

Suburban –Working in the outlining areas of a large metropolitan city can be filled with opportunities. To start, a larger number of cases may have HMOs because households are likely to have at least one parent working. There may also be more people wanting to be seen in the evening and on Saturdays so they won't have to miss work. So you may have to be creative in meeting their needs. But remember that you will have to wait at 50 to 66 days to get reimbursement for your services.

Rural - Rural communities require more development and travel time. You may drive two hours or more to reach just one of the communities you serve. You may even find that you have to stay overnight in order to see enough patients. Of course, there is less competition for cases in rural communities, but it will cost you more money to service those cases. If you consider the cost of gasoline and the wear and tear on your vehicle, the costs of staying in a hotel or motel for at least two nights and the additional costs of eating out, you quickly realize that you are spending a lot just to be able to work in these communities.

If an established organization hires a part-time therapist, the therapist will demand at least 40% more in reimbursement, mileage, lodging and support costs. If you travel 160 miles to and from a rural community, the mileage reimbursement rate will pay about $120 and the motel for two nights can easily be another $160. If you are paying a part-time therapist $30 per hour in a metropolitan area and they bill 20 in three days of work, they are making $600 and the organization is receiving $440, given the Medicaid rate of reimbursement. If the organization pays for the motel and mileage then that $440 becomes $160. If you have to pay an additional 20% to the part time therapist then you could be losing another $120, and now it's costing you $40 a week above what you receive in reimbursement. This situation makes it nearly impossible to make money servicing rural communities in this way, and without grant funding it's impossible to operate in the red for any length of time.

The costs of operating in the rural community are significant, and Medicaid and Medicare need to re-evaluate their reimbursement rates for rural mental health organizations. There is a critical shortage of mental health specialists in the rural communities, especially along the borders. The low rate of reimbursement, the lack of adequate health care infrastructure, the priorities of the political hierarchy and the foundations that follow the political gods all contribute to the higher operating costs and the critical shortage of healthcare providers.

Marketplace Obstacles

There is a growing lack of resources for those who need medical and mental health services. It has been estimated that "22.1 percent of Americans ages 18 and older – about 1 in 5 adults – suffer from a diagnosable mental disorder in a given year. When applied to the 1998 U. S. Census residential population estimate, this figure translates to 44.3 million people. In addition, 4 of the 10 leading causes of disability in the U.S. and other developed countries are mental disorders – major depression, bipolar, schizophrenia, and obsessive-compulsive disorder." (National Institute of Mental Health, 2004, p. 1).

The numbers of mentally ill children in crisis also appears to be at record levels. For example, in the Greater Cincinnati area there have been more "ill children admitted to the psychiatric unit at Children's Hospital Medical Center than to any similar hospital in the country in 2002." (The Enquirer, 2004 p. 1) In Los Angeles several emergency rooms have been closed. "Across the state, 70 emergency departments and trauma centers have closed since 1990. Of Los Angeles County's nine million residents, 30% are underinsured or uninsured, according to Carol Meyer, director of the Los Angeles County Emergency Medical Services Agency. The state's 500 hospitals are 'on the verge of a whole series of unraveling events,' Dr. Jack Lewin, the executive director of

CMA has reported, and 'there's no one to pay for it.'" (Kaisernetwork. org, 8/21/04)

In a 2003 survey the House Committee on Government Reform surveyed 524 juvenile detention centers nationwide and found that 33 states detained children with mental illnesses who faced no criminal charges. Also the report found that of the 2,000 children with mental illness in detention centers remain incarcerated because of a lack of access to treatment. In addition, the report found that many were younger than age eleven. (Kaisernetwork.org, 1/8/04)

In the midst of this crisis, Medicaid cuts have caused people of all ages to suffer needlessly. According to a statement attributed to James Scully, Jr., M.D., Medical Director, American Psychiatric Association, Richard Birkel, Ph.D., Executive Director, National Allianced for the Mentally Ill, and Michael Faenza, MSSW, President, National Mental Health Association, "restricting access to needed services and medications only forces people with mental disorders on Medicaid into hospital emergency rooms and jails, which are now saddled with providing costly and inappropriate care for people with mental illnesses.

Many states that have slashed Medicaid are now experiencing the disastrous aftermath. The emergency room at Massachusetts General Hospital saw a 40 percent increase in psychiatric patients from April 2002 to April 2003. At a hospital in Columbia, SC, two emergency room lobbies were converted recently into waiting areas after some 20 people a day sought psychiatric care and overwhelmed the mental health unit. In fact, emergency facilities are so overtaxed that a recent federal report indicated that they are not 'boarding' patients – an unprecedented phenomenon." (nmha.org, 4/4/04)

Over 82 million U.S. residents under 65 years of age have been uninsured at some point during the years of 2002 and 2003, a dramatic increase over the rate of 74.7 million the previous year. African

Americans and Hispanics are the most likely uninsured, with nearly 60% of Hispanics and 43% of American Americans lacking coverage at some point during the study period. In addition, it has been reported that among families with incomes of at least $75,000, 13.5 million were without insurance for part of the 2002-2003 (Congress Daily, 6/16) In fourteen states, more than one-third of the non-elderly population was without health insurance during at least part of the study period (USA Today 6/16). Texas had the highest uninsured rate in the United States, with 43.4% of residents under 65 without coverage at some point during the study period." (kaisernetwork.org, 6/18/04)

Now there is a growing shortage of services due, in part, to overloading of emergency rooms, but also due to an increasing shortage of nurses, physicians, and mental health professionals in rural and border-to-border counties (along the border with Mexico from California to Texas). For example, the shortage of nurses has resulted from increased requirements for accreditation of hospitals and some group practices by the Joint Commission of Accreditation, the downsizing of hospitals, nurses leaving more traditional nursing positions and becoming Nurse Practitioners or administrators, and the aging of the workforce. Texas alone is facing a shortage of 40,000 nurses, but the shortage is nationwide. (www.uthscsa.edu, 4/18/04)

There is also a shortage of physicians. The report in the *San Antonio Business Journal* stated that the Texas Medical Association claims that deep cuts in "state funds and steadily decreasing federal funds for graduate medical education are colliding with an aging population that needs more care than ever. Limits on hours that physicians in training can work, and huge numbers of uninsured patients at hospital emergency rooms are exacerbating the problem. 'If Texas doesn't train the next generation of doctors here, they'll go to another state for their residences,' says Dr. Roland Goertz, a Waco doctor and chairman of the TMA Committee on Physician Distribution and Health Care Access." (www.bizjournals.com, 6/14/04) While this represents Texas' problems, it would appear to be similar in other states, too based on other articles.

Assessing the Needs of a Selected Population

If you are working within a community that either has very little need for your services or has an overabundance of providers, your caseload will be meager. If you work within a community where people do not believe in psychology or mental health, you may not get many referrals. Therefore, it pays to study the mental health needs of a community as well as its prominent belief systems. Talk to therapists, psychologists, psychiatrists, primary care physicians, school counselors and hospital social workers or other administrators. Talk to rabbis, chaplains, priests or ministers. Even speak with real estate agents—they will give you information about how the city or town is growing and where new schools are likely to be built next. The more information you have, the better.

Get to know your competition: what organizations are working in the area, what insurance companies are selling policies in the community, etc. Check out the local business community; ask about their health insurance and then complete application for representation with those insurance companies. If a large percentage of the community has Blue Cross/Blue Shield (Blue), find out what policies they have(e.g., governmental, state, Border Patrol, school district, Blue Choice, Blue First, etc.). Knowing this ahead of time can help you know what Blue panel you need to get on. Just because you have been accepted on one Blue panel doesn't automatically qualify you for all Blue panels. The sources mentioned in the last paragraph can probably give you much of the information you need to determine if you want to work in that community or with that population, or if you want to go to another community across town.

There are disparities between metro and rural communities in regards to income and education levels. These factors are often associated with differences in the occurrence of illness and death, including heart disease, diabetes, obesity, elevated blood lead levels, and low birth weights. Higher incomes permit an increase in access to medical and mental health specialists and more group support programs. Physicians may not accept Medicaid or patients with no income, but they seldom pass on a cash patient.

രുജ്

Case Study

This case illustrates one example of the obstacles facing those with limited resources living in rural communities. Maria is a 24-year-old Hispanic married female who is still waiting to become a naturalized citizen after being brought to Del Rio by her parents when she was only 6 years old. When her parents came to Texas from Mexico their legal representative told them that they could not include the family in the application for naturalization. Only the father and mother were included. There is a twelve-year wait for legal residency for most applicants. After Maria got married she made an application. That was four years ago. She is still waiting. In the meantime she can not afford to go through a border patrol inspection center because she has no legal status even though her parents brought to America. If she went to San Antonio without the special authorization from a Mexican consulate (such as for medical care) she can expect that the authorities would attempt to deport her back to Mexico. Since she was brought to America by her father and mother without a passport, she has no proof that she a Mexican citizen. Therefore, she is a woman without a country until her application gets approved (which might take another ten years). This is only one case that illustrates some of the problems of living along the border and living daily with fear of being arrested, separated from your family and deported. You don't see this type of case every day but it documents some of the conditions people are either living in or fear of living in. For others, they share addresses in the United States with others but live in Mexico so their children can go to school in America. They fear being discovered and their fears and anxieties are passed onto their children.

CR80

Economic Level of Practice Population

The economic level of your practice population can indicate the types of disorders you might see, the types of educational backgrounds you patients are likely to have, and the family traditions and beliefs that may reflect on their views of the world. It can also tell you something about their problems, their expectations of you and what they want from you. When you compare people who expect their doctor to be available to them 24/7 to someone who expects to have to wait for a couple of weeks to get an appointment to talk to you, you may choose one over the other. If you don't want patients to call you at all hours, don't ever call them on your cell phone. Instead, have an answering service that can connect you if you have to talk to them in an emergency. During the first session, have your staff explain to your new patients about how calls are handled, and that if they don't show up for appointment they may be charged a fee. If they have an insurance policy that will not reimburse this fee, or forbids any charges in addition to those charged for specific services, you have the right to fire them as patients.

If you work in a community or with a population that expects to "drop in" and "drop out" without consideration to your busy schedule or the costs of an "empty" time slot to you, then you might as well add another 30% to your costs. If your cost to operate one office for a month is $90,000 (including your salary and that of your receptionist), then 30% would translate into $27,000. Most communities have people who qualify for Medicaid or SCHIPS. These generally offer the lowest reimbursement rates for medical or mental health services. Sometimes an EAP will offer you $30 or $40 when everyone else is paying $50 or more per hour. If you fill your practice with the lowest rates, you will have to work longer to make the money that others are receiving. On the other hand, in the past Medicaid has reimbursed faster then most HMOs and with less paperwork requirements. However, this appears to be changing. At one time Medicaid didn't have many providers, so the states allowed for less interference from the administrators. Gradually, over time and due to different budget priorities, new managed care procedures for being seen by a health care provider and an increase in accessibility are driving up the costs of health care practices, because more people are going to receive medical care for their children. One reason is that schools will not accept children who have not had all their recommended shots.

Every time an insurance company requires more paperwork justification, asks for additional phone calls for pre-authorization, lengthens the time it takes to receive reimbursement, or cuts the number of therapy sessions, they are increasing the costs of doing business for providers. Do some simple mathematical calculations: to pull a chart for review or for the preparation of another insurance form or/and telephonic message or conversation is a minimum of 15 minutes. Most case managers in workers' compensation use this time calculation. If your practice costs you $15,000 a month to keep the doors open, and you only work 160 hours a month, then 15 minutes translates into $23.44. Even if your staff fills out the forms and you only have to read it and sign it, it doesn't matter. You still must have your staff stop doing some other task to handle the paperwork. And you have to stop seeing people in order to read, correct and then sign the form. If your practice has only three therapists, and each has 5 of these forms or phone interruptions or pre-authorizations per week, that translates into 60 per month, which is $1,406 in expenses you cannot bill for, thus increasing your overhead by nearly 10%. To make up this amount money you have to increase your billable hours by 4 per week. That's working an additional hour per day four days a week for four weeks, or working two Saturdays per month, just to pay for additional paperwork or/and phone calls for patients' insurance companies regarding your cases. You can probably safely bet that the insurance companies are not letting their people work an extra hour or day a week because of problems with a union or because they don't want to pay overtime rates. But they don't mind asking you to spend extra time and/or money to do something so you can basically stay in business. What other industry could do this legally?

In different cities around America there are small groups of physicians, therapists, chiropractors and perhaps others who are running cash-only businesses. Others are doing retainer businesses. A retainer may be $5,000, or for a family $10,000, and then the doctors agree to be responsive to calls for the year on an hourly basis. If you have an emergency you call your doctor at 4:30 a.m. and he/she will promise to answer the phone. These doctors and therapists promise to spend as much time as their clients need to help decrease the pain or/and symptoms. This is a growing and exciting alternative to having to wait two hours to see a doctor for ten minutes. You would not try this in a rural community because patients often are much more accustomed to just showing up, some as early as 6 a.m. and are willing to wait. When you start seeing patients many will have waited several hours. Knowing the population you want to serve can save you a lot of grief and financial problems later.

Developing Mission and Vision Statements

It can be very useful to write mission and vision statements for your practice to help keep focused as well as a way of marketing your services. A vision statement is a written declaration of an organization's valiant plan to do some gallant task for the common good.. It is general in nature and lacks specifics. An example is the Texas Department of Mental Health and Mental Retardation's (MHMR) vision: "The mental health and mental retardation system will be a partnership of consumers, family members, service providers and policy makers which creates options responsive to individual needs and preferences." (Texas, 2004, p. 1)

A mission statement describes how your organization is going to reach its vision.. This statement is more specific, not as grandiose. The Texas MHMR mission statement is: "To improve the quality and efficiency of public and private services and supports for Texans with mental illnesses and with mental retardation so that they can increase their opportunities and abilities to lead lives of dignity and independence." (Texas MHMR, 2004, p. 1)

Developing a Business Plan

Organizations use strategic planning sessions to determine what the organization is going to sell, who is going to purchase the product or service, how the products or services will be delivered to the public, who is going to perform the services or make the products, where the products will be made or where the services will be performed, when is this plan going to start and when will this plan be re-evaluated.

A business plan makes a number of assumptions. For example, the plan might assume that, with "x" number of dollars might buy your organization "n" number of staff, hire "x" number of professionals and offer "y" number of new programs in order to see "z" number of patients. Another assumption may be that this practice will continue to grow. This assumption may be based on your past experience, or you may believe it because some book told you to expect this result or because you have statistics from the local health district regarding the number of people who accessed medical and mental health services. Assumptions tell your banker how you will address business problems within your practice. They also serve, for you, as a road map to where you are going and how you plan on dealing with the roadblocks.

Medical Model vs. Problem Solving

A business plan for your banker will describe what you are selling and how much it will cost and how much you will be paid for your time. Selling your product (herbal supplements) or service (chiropractic adjustments, medical evaluations and treatment, psychological evaluations, psychotherapy, etc.) to the public will be different from selling it to your banker. Presentation, terms, figures will differ depending on your audience. You present a business plan to the banker because you want money to expand your services. You are explaining what the goals of the organization are and how you will reach them. You are problem solving. In order to increase your practice you can make a brochure for potential patients and distribute them to community outlets (schools, other health care provider offices, stores, etc.).

Physicians, chiropractors and physical therapists operate more from a medical therapeutic model rather then a problem-solving model because their cases look for biological and genetic etiologies first, mental health secondary. Mental health therapists work in reverse, studying medical, social, family, and educational histories first before exploring physical causes. Practicing under a "medical model" is something physicians have worked on for years, and managed care has demanded a "medical need" for justification for treatment. Psychologists and therapists from different disciplines are forced to use this model in order to receive reimbursement; however, it may lead to some type of semantically disagreement or incongruency because these therapists are more likely to use a cognitive-behavioral approach to a problem solving issue. Most insurance companies expect this type of approach due to research literature. But it may still cause another obstacle to reimbursement. The medical model's assumption is that the patient is "sick" and can't help him/herself. Patients view themselves as victims who need help someone to solve their problems. "It's not MY fault," or "I can't do anything, I'm disabled. I have ADHD and I only have a GED. I can't even get a job!"

Psychotherapists today tend to help patients find ways they can overcome their physical "disorders" and learning or emotional disabilities. This approach states: "You are not helpless, and I will work and stay with you until you learn the techniques to overcome these problems." Those providers who work to empower patients by recognizing their responsibility for their own behavior without calling them "bad" or "sick." Each person has the answer to their problems but may benefit from dialoguing with an objective and trained therapist who has training and appreciation of the biological, chemical and genetic factors of a given mental health issue. Framing a problem in this way can help a patient gain insight into his/her own strength levels.

"Eliminating the medical model does not eliminate consideration of biological, chemical, or genetic issues. For example, some people may be genetically determined to be more drawn to alcohol than others. Is this fair? It doesn't matter. These people must find the resources to respond emotionally, psychologically, and behaviorally to this challenge, or else they become stuck in their problems without much hope. To excuse people from this responsibility is an act of disempowerment. Medical model thinking disarms people in ways from which many never recover." (Ackley, 1997, p. 52) While physicians use the medical model, psychotherapists have options.

Mental health and social work therapists and counselors, including drug and alcohol counselors, have been using alternatives to the medical model for years with a lot of success. These therapists are dealing with guiding patients through dis-ease (an uncomfortable feeling like feeling off-balance) as well as disease and disorders. The end result is also different then the medical model. A physician sets a broken arm and it heals. A social worker helps a family find resource within the community and the family resolves their own problems. A therapist helps a couple find ways to work their way through a tragic loss in their lives. We all do valuable things, and we need to tell people about those things. This may mean changing how we talk to them and how we word what we do on a brochure or during a community presentation.

Developing a Sales Plan

Developing a sales plan is a marketing strategy to determine how the product will be sold to the identified consumers or distributors. Marketing a health care organization is the process of networking and advertising. The marketers, or maybe just the owner or provider if it's a one person operation or a small group, will make brochures and business cards and take them to primary care physicians, dentists, medical specialists, internists, physical therapists, chiropractors, ministers, rabbis, priests, school counselors, other mental health care providers, other small businesses, and radio and television studios. Often the radio and television studios will interview you, especially in small communities.

Metropolitan communities may have a radio station that will interview you, but unless you promise to have sex with a patient, or say something outrageous (like too much sun can cause paranoia), most television stations will ignore you. In small rural communities the local radio station is the primary source of community information.

Brochures should be attractive and should look professional. There are software programs that can guide you through this process. However, you will probably want to be trained by an "expert" first. Many people don't have time to read the instructions or don't have time to translate them into "common" English. For me it still means a lot of trial and error time. Be sure to answer several key questions in your advertisements. What are you going to sell? Mental health services? What type? Marital therapy, biofeedback, psychotherapy, group therapy? For what type of issues? Depression, panic attacks, nerves? Do I have to be crazy to see you? Will my insurance cover what you do? Do I have to lie on a couch? Will you make me cry? How long do I have to keep seeing you? Explain to me again why I want to see you?

Power Point

Building your practice means making it to withstand the onslaught of liabilities and costs of doing business. It means building a practice that uses techniques, structure, policies and procedures that reflect a defensive policy and an appreciation of risks. Although you may have a heart of gold, the patience of Job, and the wisdom of Solomon, you could lose your life, your practice, and your home if you fail to build wisely (legal structure, infrastructure, financing) and install certain safety fixtures (self-audits, compliance policies, and billing policies).

CX80

End of Chapter Review

Multiple Choices Questions

1. What type of practice is one that ten therapists working for one employer?
    a. Private Practice
    b. Group Practice
    c. Contract Practice
    d. MHMR

2. What type of practice may not require a state license?
    a. Private Practice
    b. Group Practice
    c. Contract Practice
    d. MHMR

3. What type of practice requires professional liability insurance?
    a. Private Practice
    b. Group Practice
    c. Contract Practice
    d. All the above

4. How can low social-economic factors affect your practice?
    a. Predominance of HMOs
    b. Non-compliance and a increase in no shows
    c. An increase in professional liability premiums
    d. You'll need a translator
    e. All the above

5. What type of practice many be the most expensive to operate?
    a. Rural
    b. Suburban
    c. Urban
    d. Contract

Rethink

1. Explain how personal research can help your practice.

2. Discuss the advantages to working near your home.

3. Discuss the value of a sales plan.

4. Write a vision statement.

5. Write a mission statement.

Personal Observation Exercise

1. Go the Internet and lookup the Texas Secretary of State Report of at www.secretaryofstate.tx.us. Compare the data of those communities who are classified as metropolitan counties and those who are classified as rural or/and border counties.

2. Talk to a nurse in a local doctor office and ask about shortages and opportunities in the local health care community.

Chapter Seven
Developing An Infrastructure For
A Multi-Specialty Practice

Summary

Infrastructure is vital for the adequate administration and deliver of health care services to a community. If you are the only health care provider in the county, it will be difficult to refer patients to specialists or primary care physicians who may be able to collaborate on a case. Seldom is a disease of the body not a dis-ease for the mind. Having other professionals available with reasonable driving distance can be crucial to the success, even the survival, of a practice.

You learn in this chapter:

1. How infrastructure affects the quality of health care.
2. How infrastructure can improve the quality of life of members of a community.
3. Types of professional licenses and professional services that might improve the quality of your practice.
4. The importance of external audits to a practice.
5. The value of a compliance policy and committee.

The Framework

The term "infrastructure" may or may not be a frequent visitor to your vocabulary store. It can often be a somewhat confusing and mysterious term. In the early years of this world after Adam and Eve, people roamed to places that offered food and water and temporary shelter. They lived in caves, drank from streams, and hunted near their cave. When they decided to stay longer in one place, they began to be concerned with cultivating crops. To plant seeds they needed some type of tool. Since they probably didn't have a Sears, Penny's or Wards department stores, and they certainly didn't have a Wal-Mart, they had to create the tool. Then they needed supplies to build the tools they needed. They needed seeds to plant, and they needed a way to get water closer to their cave and crops. These early needs suggest the beginning of a community infrastructure. Today our cities have constructed maintained and supported roads, sewage and water supplies for those in the community. An infrastructure supports human needs, primarily economic but it also includes religious, political, educational, social and cultural. Roads lead to hospitals and stores, schools and work places. Telephone system supports communication between the denizens. Sewage and water are needed to support good health. Buses, trains, airlines support the movement of people and merchandise with outside communities. Buildings are built to support office space, small business entrepreneurs, big businesses, chamber of commerce, city public services, police and fire departments, city hall, gas stations, city tax assessor, entertainment centers and convention halls.

One definition of infrastructure is the physical facilities which move people (transportation, roads, airlines, buses, trains, etc.) and commodities (food, furniture, manufacturing goods etc.), utilities, waste, energy and information (ITT, cable, telephone, phones, etc.). The basic goal of infrastructure is about delivering goods and services that help in the formation of basic support systems that is used to provide the delivery of goods and services more effective and efficient. Another explanation "ties together different strands of legal and economic thought pertaining to natural resources such as lakes, traditional infrastructure such as road system, what antitrust theorists describe as essential facilities, basic scientific research and the Internet." (1)

The Illinois State Chamber of Commerce states that "infrastructure is an essential foundation of our business community with far reaching impact across all strata of our state and society." (2) They go on to point out how infrastructure is used for the common good thus fulfilling the Chambers' mission.

Infrastructure has been defined in more economical terms, but it can be applied to medical and mental health organizations in communities that need health services at some point(s) of their lives, including the lives of their family. But it can be described in terms of choices. An infrastructure provides choices for the community. You can go to the movies or stay home and watch a DVD. You can go eat in one side of town, or go the other side for dinner, even travel to another city. You have the choice of flying to another state for a week-end or longer. You can get on the Internet and search for information about your favorite team that is 3,000 miles away.

In terms of the health profession, infrastructure can bring choices to the business community and to the citizens of that community. With roads that are big enough to hold eighteen wheelers you have the potential of bringing any type of goods and services to that community. With a hospital in the community you have the ability of attract other health care services. With schools you attract families. But if your roads are breaking down you have problems getting trucks to the community. Without rail no train will go through the city or county. Without cell phone towers cell phones are no good. When the community spends more time on congested roads they spend less time at home with their families. After a while the families will talk about moving. "We need to establish a comprehensive, long-term infrastructure plan as opposed to our current 'patch and pray' method to ensure a better quality of life for everyone," states William P. Henry, P.E., President, American Society of Civil Engineers (ASCE). (3) The investment needed for protecting our current infrastructure is controlled by the Department of Homeland Security. Who defines the use of the health care finances? Congress use has contracted the MCOs and HMOs to administer the fund through filters and obstacles of health care..

A few weeks after the 9-11-01 tragedy in New York City and Washington, D.C., Ken Chamberlain, President and CEO, National Mental Health Association told a congressional committee: "The nation needs to understand that we are woefully unprepared for the mental health ramifications of the disasters, which we can expect to emerge. The medical evidence is clear that the unpredictable acts of malice along with protracted recovery efforts lead to a higher incidence of mental health problems. An uncertainty of what the future will hold adds to the nation's level of stress." (4) Almost four years since "ground zero" billions have gone into attacking and defending against terrorist threats and acts. Much of that has come from health care programs.

Infrastructure is vital to any practice of health care because infrastructure is the framework within which operates the professional core. Licensed professionals are the core of the practice of health care because without them there can not be any legal entity called health care. Ingredients of an infrastructure includes a place to practice, personnel to do administrative and clerical work, bookkeeper and Certified Professional Accountant (CPA) to perform tax accountability including preparation and filing, a place to store files securely and safely, para-professionals to perform to assist the professionals with key tasks, key specialists to perform human resource duties, grant writing, compliance duties, quality assurance audits, and business development. Experienced and knowledgeable personnel are needed for pre-authorization, billing and collections. A legal team needs experienced in corporate law, copyright laws, professional liability, contract law, and criminal law.

In any productive organization the chain of command is the stablizer of the organization. Normally there is a senior professional who is selected (by vote or by the one with the most financial investment or/and senior partner) as a President or/and CEO of the practice. The professionals then select an Executive Director or Administrator to run the operation of practice. In a smaller groups where there are not enough funds to hire an Administrator, an Office Manager often is responsible for administrative duties. An Office Manager is the office cop, directing traffic at the front office, setting appointments, pulling charts, making sure that the doctors or therapists are busy seeing people, answering questions, ensuring the timely answering of phones, sending faxes, doing dictation and pre-authorization of insurance coverage. An Office Manager usually is doing many of these tasks, where as the Administrator supervises these tasks and is more involved in writing office policies and procedures, ensuring HIPPA compliance and hiring and terminating, and ensuring that the professionals obtain the continuing education credits there licenses require. They also represent the practice at compliance related conferences and seminars. He/She does many of the human resource tasks in place of a human resource professional/specialist.

Non-profit organizations may qualify for funding from governmental agencies and non-profit foundations. Being a non-profit organization changes the frame work, therefore, some of the staff requirements. More about non-profit organizations will be discussed in another chapter. Also, a community MHMR organization will be discussed in another chapter.

A Community Mental Health Center is a designation by the state to incorporate mental health services within the frame work of a regulated state program. Those Centers who operate under this designation can get funding from the state that other mental health organizations can not.

Types Of Licenses Needed

Types of licensed professionals needed are determined by the type of practice: medical, mental health, social service agency, physical or/and occupational, chiropractic, or rehabilitation practice. The practice can start as one type of practice and expand to include other services and programs offered. As each service is offered, a parallel search is done of the laws of the state and also of Medicaid, Medicare and the HMOs the practice represents. When an investment is made to hire a Nurse Practitioner or the clinic administrator wants to expand services there are certain billing and legal hurdles. For example, Medicaid can take up to 6 months to approve a billing number for a new therapist, doctor, or nurse. If a medical clinic wants to offer physical rehabilitation there may be some restrictions for medical doctors referring to themselves. Can a non-licensed professional set-up a medical clinic? If a medical doctor agrees to perform the medical duties, is it possible, but a license will not be issued unless you have an agreement in writing. In Texas licensed professionals that can bill Medicaid, Medicare and HMOs include medical doctors, family nurse practitioners, physician assistants, psychiatrists, chiropractors, clinical psychologists, licensed professional counselors, licensed marriage and family therapists, licensed social workers, registered physical therapists, occupational therapists, dentists, eye clinics, massage therapists, licensed vocational nurses,

Staff Skill Positions

Support staffs included receptionists, insurance clerk (pre-authorization, billing and collections), data base clerk, accounts payable, office manager, business developer or marketing representative, computer specialist (on contract), and legal (on retainer or as needed).

One of the pressing issues of a new therapist is who to hire for office support. There isn't any standard for quality of for a biller of insurance HCFA forms. There is no requirement that they have a degree or a certification. If they are over or under bill a case, it is **your** fault. That may be the only standard although you will find people that have lots of experience but who only want to bill as an outsource. Most people don't have the investment to hire and develop an office manager or a billing staff until they become proficient. Therefore, ask other professionals what and who they recommend, then take their advice.

છ૪૦

Case Study:

A therapist hired someone he could afford. She paid her near minimum wage. After a year working in the office she made a mistake on a HCFA form. The biller carefully whited it out with liquid white-out, and then sent the bills to the HMO. Somehow the bill was questioned and the therapist called her attorney. The therapist's attorney recommended hiring an exterior auditor. The therapist agreed. The auditor was hired by the attorney and came in and audited not only the HMO's cases but others randomly. The auditor went to the HMO with the therapist and explained what had happened and handed them a check for the over-billed part. The HMO determined that there was no intent to defraud them and they accepted the check of $850. The auditor's fee and the attorney's fee amounted to $20,000.

Did the therapist do the right thing? Why? Could this mistake be foreseen or prevented?

CRRO

Administrator or Office Manager - An Office Manager usually is less experienced then an administrator, and is paid less. An Office Manager usually is involved in many of the tasks of running an office. An Administrator will focus on Human Resource, Code and HIPPA compliance, and handling office communications, training and development and puts out the "office fires".

Telephone Coverage - A pleasant and professional telephone voice is critical to a practice because people are calling because they are having emotional problems with their life or someone important to them. It is important that the receptionist is friendly and can connect with those on the phone. At the same time the receptionist needs to draw boundaries. It is not the job of the receptionist to discuss the patient's problems. That is the job of the therapist or physician. Getting information such as, why are they calling now? What insurance coverage do they have and is it current? And when can they come in? Finally, checking their current phone number can be very important. People change phone numbers; sometimes they use a message phone. If you have to change their appointment before they come in, not being able to reach them can cause a lot of problems for them and the office.

The receptionist is a critical front line of defense for an office. The friendly but professional voice and presentation helps with patients and vendors as well as with other professionals who call you or other health care providers.

Answering the phone by the third ring can be very reassuring for the callers. It decreases their anxiety and reassures the caller that they are closer to having their problem solved and their pain decreased.

An answering service or Notes system can be helpful for catching messages not caught during the day or after hours. Someone needs to pick-up and answer all calls before the office closes and first thing the next workday morning preferably during the first hour.

Pre-authorizations – An Office Manager handles pre-authorizations. In a small office an Office Manger often does the billings and collections. When the Office Manager is overwhelmed, things get bottled up, which means billings not getting out quickly and revenues streams being low and slow. If pre-authorizations are not done, you can be seeing people for free because some companies will not pay for what they do not authorize. And even then, companies have refused payment which causes delays and additional paperwork and possible legal action. Costs add up quicker then you can blink.

Billing and Collections – Billings and collections is critical for keeping the doors open. If you don't know how to bill you can hire someone or outsource it to a specialist. Knowledge is king in billing and collections. You can bill thousands of dollars but if your billing codes are out of date, or if you are billing for something you can not bill for, collections will not come in as expected or needed. Billing records and the ageing of the receivables is critical in forecasting and monitoring your office receivables. Not keeping good records can lead to wrong impressions and it is hard to verify something that doesn't exist. You may think you should be having $9,000 come in next month but it may be only $5,900 because of a lack of timely pre-authorizations or insurance policies not being enforce a particular month.

Data Base Clerk – A data base is a file with important and relevant information regarding your patients. Collection of various histories, such as medical, social, mental health, educational, number of children, marital status, number of sessions per diagnosis or/and year, different DSM-IVR codes used in treatment, and any referrals for psychological evaluations, psychiatric evaluation, medication evaluation, and/or referral to a hospital. The individual performing the data base entries is responsible for following the directions of the professional staff (usually a committee) in performing data entry, then pulling out the information into an organized fashion that is designed by the professional staff and the computer contractor or specialist. The written reports are usually pulled out within 5 days of the end of the month and presented to the Office Manager or Administrator who is responsible for presentation to the professional staff.

If an organization is funded by non-profit or/and governmental agencies, the collection base is likely to quite lengthy in order to support evaluation and research requirements.

Bookkeeping – If you have a small office (just yourself or a couple of employees); you are probably going to handle the accounts' payable. In larger groups it may pay to have an outside firm that offers a wide variety of services including tax returns, financial analysis, bookkeeping, payment to vendors, and retirement programs. The can also assist with financial forecasting and needs assessment. It can be very helpful to have their reports when you visit your banker.

Banking – Having a banker that you can build up a relationship with can help you when you need a Line of Credit. This is a revolving line of credit that must be paid down in order to get more money. It is usually secured on office furniture, or on accounts receivable. It's not a typical loan where you pay-off then, to get more money you complete another application. A Line of Credit means if you have $25,000 and you take out $5,000, you can write a check for up to $20,000. As you pay it off, you can write checks for the difference between the balance and $25,000 without completing another application.

Having a banker that understands the type of business you are in can speed up loans that you might need, i.e., car, equipment, payroll, etc. There are general business cycles that affects most big businesses then there are seasonal adjustments for smaller businesses, i.e., slower during certain months or times of the year. For example, if you are working with children, and you visit them in the schools, you will not be able to see them at schools during vacations, holidays, summer months, or testing periods.

Last year one school district that I visited figured that they were testing 80% of the time. This can cause problems when attempting to develop a relationship with your patients in order to encourage behavioral change. If the school doesn't want their students being interrupted at school, then the parent must bring them to the office. If the parent has trouble getting the child to the office on a regular basis because they have so many commitments to work or after school projects or programs, or the mother doesn't have transportation. If there is a medical need for mental health or medical care, then the parent can be charged with medical neglect by Child Protective Services. In addition, if you notify their insurance company, some, like Medicaid, will either call the parent or tell them to find a way to have their child seen, or they could loose medical or mental health services for that particular diagnosis. Many parents believe that all they have to do is get their child diagnosed and they can apply for SSI benefits. But more disability judges will look at the services or the lack of them, as an important part of his/her decision. Medication alone is not always accepted as an adequate attempt to resolve their problems.

Committees And Professional Duties

Compliance Committee Membership - In a small organization the only people that may be available for this committee is the owner, clinical director and the Office Manager. But in larger practices the owner or senior officer is NOT on this committee. A Compliance Officer is designated along with members representing the professional staff as well as the billing department and/or Administrator. They meet monthly and a report is kept of meeting minutes. If the professional staff has weekly, ethical concerns may be presented as well as questions regarding billing codes or procedures. These can then be forwarded to the Compliance Officer who will ensure that the next meeting cover these concerns and then the Compliance Officer will get back to the next professional staff meeting with a report on the committee's discussion and conclusions if any. There may be a request from the Compliance Committee to consult with the organization's legal team to get an opinion. These types of actions are not only a good way to support a healthy practice, but also to encourage professional ethics. It is also a solid formula for documenting INTENTION to comply with state, federal and HMO's rules and regulations. As will be discussed in another chapter (Liabilities) when there is an investigation of insurance fraud, investigators have to prove INTENT to defraud. When you can prove that over time the organization, the professionals within the practice, actively promote ways to discover (internal discussion and audits) as well as yearly or bi-annual external audits, the argument about the intent to defraud grows harder to defend.

Any practice would be smart to develop a compliance policies and procedures manual. Even if there is only one physician or therapist the manual will be proof of intentions of the owner to follow the rules and regulations.

a. Compliance of regulations and grant awards – If there are contracts and grants that are awarded, there will be a requirement that the organization be accountable for the funds, and that there be an assessment process to monitor the allotment of funding to ensure that the funds pays for what the granting or contracting agency requires. There will also be a requirement that the organization providing the required services also have an evaluation form or survey that provides feedback from patients or families serviced as to the amount of satisfaction they had of those services.

b. Quality Assurance Audits - Medicaid, Medicare and HMOs have a program to periodically review every provider to ensure quality of services. You might not see one for five or six years then they may show up and ask to review x number of files. Usually they will provide a list of names and will ask your staff to pull those charts and then provide a room and desk where they can review the files in private. The disruption to your staff and practice is a cost of doing business.

President, Chief Executive Officer (CEO), Executive Director – In a one-person practice, the titles are not particularly important. If the individual incorporates, usually a Sub S corporation, there is the requirement for a least two officers. Shares of the stock normally stay with one person. For larger practices, there may be a President, Vice-President, Secretary-Treasurer, or the President may also be the CEO and instead of a VP there may be a Chief Operating Officer (COO). Normally a non-profit organization will hire an Executive Director who acts as the CEO and organizational spokesman for the organization. The senior officer is the one that sets the tone, the attitude and the direction of the organization. This officer often works with a Board of Directors and a committee of officers to manage, challenges and directs the priorities and objectives through a quagmire of legal, accountability and community responsibilities. The CEO works with his team, and the legal and banking contacts to protect the organization against legal and fiscal assaults.

Compliance Officer – COO or Clinical Director of the practice. Chairs the Compliance Committee. The Compliance Officer must have authority and senior management responsibility in order to enforce compliance to committee recommendations. Next to a corporate attorney this committee can do more to protect an organization against legal actions.

Clinical Director – Usually a senior psychologist or therapist who supervises the clinical staff and makes annual employee performance feedback. In a group practice of physicians this position is called Medical Director.

Program Director – Develops relevant programs the professionals and para-professionals can administer. Then evaluates the quality and satisfaction of the programs. Coordinates with the COO, VP or CEO on the type of programs the organization wants to offer the communities where its influence reaches.

Human Resource Manager – In a larger group practice a Human Resource Manager may be needed. Usually the small practice the owner fills this position. In small group practice an Office Manager may share some of these tasks. In a larger practice an Administer handles human resources responsibilities. But when the group has multi-specialists and perhaps multiple cites, a human resource manager, with 3 – 5 years of experience can be hired to keep the practice in line with all local, state and federal laws and regulations regarding the hiring, training, and termination of personnel, professional, para-professionals and staff.

Legal Resources - A small practice normally can not afford adequate legal representation. However, hiring an attorney who has experience in health care law can help you with ethical and legal issues of a normal practice. The attorney can guide you through the development of a Compliance Manual and can hire an outside auditor for your annual or bi-annual audits.

For larger organizations the following legal coverage is a necessity:

a. Corporation
b. Patient/Trade Mark
c. Professional Liability

    d. Contracts

    e. Criminal

<u>Certified Professional Accountant</u> (CPA) – may be able to assist either a small firm or a small group practice with the following tasks:
   a. Bookkeeper tasks
   b. Tax return preparation and filing
   c. Financial management (or refer you to another specialist)
   d. IRS representation (Enlisted Agent) (or refer you to another specialist)

For a single provider practice, the provider can use Quick Books for bookkeeping, balancing the check book, and printing out financial statements. However, it still can be very helpful to have someone else file your taxes and ensure the tax returns accurately reflect your financial situation and stability.

<u>Marketing or Business Development</u> – Everyone is responsible for developing referral sources. However, in larger practices, the Marketing Representative or Business Development Manager can be the focus of such efforts and can teach others how to ask for referrals. Normally this individual works with software that can help organize the marketing and development contacts and events including important task deadlines. This individual will report to the CEO or COO.

<u>Professional Training and Development</u> – In a small practice each professional is responsible for his/her continuing education courses needed. They are also responsible for storing the certificates of completion and submitting copies when needed for their annual licensing date. In larger practices the administrator or human resource manager will organize professional training development programs for

the practice, including best practice issues for the professionals and development training for the staff personnel.

External Auditor – Consult your attorney regarding the hiring of an external auditor to provide bi-annual audits of your practice. This can be the best insurance policy you can buy to protect your practice against allegations of insurance fraud. An external auditor, who is hired by your attorney has attorney, is protected by rules of confidentiality. That means your external auditor will make recommendations to you through your attorney. It would be foolish to ignore those recommendations. If the auditor finds an irregularity, it is your responsibility to fix it and your auditor can assist you with that, including how to tell an HMO or Medicaid of an over-payment. The auditor can also make recommendations regarding:

a. Practice Policies and Procedures

b. Billings

c. Progress notes, and

d. Outsourcing services like billing and collections

External Private Practice Consultant – A consultant can perform communication audits, financial analysis, program assessments, and strategic planning for an organization. A one person practice may wish to spend a day or two getting help planning a successful practice. Like this book, a consultant can save you a lot of money, disappointments and frustration. A less expensive way is using a mentor or business coach.

Board of Directors – Normally a Sub S corporation doesn't have more than a President who also serves as Secretary-Treasurer. (Consult your attorney as each state may be different in what they require of a corporation. With larger practices there may be a Board of Officers but no Board of Directors. Still others, like a non-profit organization relies on a Board of Directors to over-see the corporate operation to ensure success and community acceptance. Grant funding foundations, including governmental agencies, normally require a Board of Directors, asking that they be named on the organizational chart or in the Grant Proposal.

Corporation Officers - Corporate Officers are generally positions for a larger group practice or a non-profit organization. Corporate officers share different tasks and responsibilities of management in the corporation. Normally they communicate daily but often have weekly meetings to share information and discuss a variety of subjects to include the budget, ethical issues, short-term goals, and "hot issues" (normally a problem facing the corporation that immediate attention).

Vendors, Transportation, IT, Expansion

Vendors are suppliers of office supplies, computer equipment and repair, fax and scanner/copier and repair, and those that sell or lease equipment, cars or vans, and training equipment and videos.

Transportation is important if you have a second location to include making home or school visits or seeing patients at medical offices at another location.

IT, or information technology, includes having the most updated computer equipment, software and training and repair when needed. These are the people that can help set up a local area network (LAN) for communication enhancement (sharing a computer network to send and receive e-mails, faxes, and memos with in the office) to include the telephone service and equipment to equip each desk with a phone system that has multiple tasks and numbers. A multiple telephone system for a small group can run $5,000 up.

Expansion occurs when the organization would benefit from having an office across town or in another town. It may not require duplication of space and equipment because much of the expertise in the organization is shared within committee meetings, staff consultations, and over the telephone and computer network. During an expansion one needs to ensure that there is a way to coordinate communications and direct the flow of referrals and feedback to the referring physicians, child protective services, etc. An answering service might be cheaper then a part-time receptionist at first. Referring source require almost instant connection for communication issues. The prompt response to patients and referring sources or to primary care physicians can be very important to future work in that community. In hiring any part-time or full-time office help, it is especially important in Border States, to have some one who speaks Spanish. Where there is a community of family from the Philippines, Japan or Viet Nam, it may be important to hire someone who speaks one of those languages, too.

Power Point

Health care providers, generally speaking, do not create enough revenue to provide for adequate professional staff, training, legal team, marketing team, and quality assurance team that are needed in many cases to create a barrier of protection between lawsuits and the practice, between hostile auditors and the practice, and between state and federal agents who task is to close the practice.

End of Chapter Review

Multiple Choice

1. According to this chapter, infrastructure is the _____ of the organization.
    a. Framework
    b. Chain of Command
    c. Heart
    d. Engine

2. Who runs the front office of a small practice?
    a. Therapist or Physician
    b. Administrator
    c. Doctor's wife
    d. Office Manager

3. Who is ultimately responsible for the design of the data base and what reports are written from the data base?
    a. Data Base Clerk
    b. Professional Staff
    c. Administrator
    d. Office Manager

4. Who is responsible for developing referrals for the practice?
    a. Professional Staff
    b. Marketing Representative
    c. Office Manage or administrator
    d. Everyone

5. In larger multi-speciality and multi-clinics, who is likely to organize training and development programs for the clinic?
    a. Office Manager
    b. Administrator or Human Resources Manager
    c. COO
    d. CEO

Rethink:

1. Explain how the chain of command is the stabilizer of a

practice.

2. Discuss the role of the senior officer of the corporation (usually a President, CEO, Executive Director).

3. Discuss why an external auditor is needed in most health care practices.

4. Discuss why location is an important issue during your first five years.

5. Discuss how a single provider can open a private practice without having to borrow money or take out a loan.

CRISO

Case Study

The first few years of practicing Juan worked with a psychiatrist in general practice with more adults then children, and larger number of those with disabilities or were over 65 years of age. He also spent time with a clinical psychologist assisting her in a chronic pain management program. Gradually his individual practice was from referrals from other physicians or contacts and he felt he had to hire a temporary billing clerk who also served as an office manager and marketing representative. When the psychologist decided to close her office and work for another institution, he went full time. Within a year Juan moved into another apartment continuing to make home visits. After 6 months or so he had enough referrals to put a newspaper ad for contract workers. He hired two. Then a few months later he hired a marketing person and decided to move the office out of his second bedroom to an office. Since most of his patients were Hispanic, and several referral sources were in the predominately Hispanic community, he choose an office in a predominately Hispanic community in San Antonio (Westside) and a low social economic community.

Within 6 months his practice was getting about 35 referrals a week, primarily from Child Protective Services, primary care physicians and Foster Care Organizations. Within another year his group was adding more staff to handle the 60 referrals a week. Soon the group had 14 therapists, 6 staff personnel, expanded into two more sections on the same floor (est. 5500 sq. feet), and had a payroll over $30,000 a month.

Going from his apartment to an office meant he had to deal with a number of infrastructure issues. Discuss possible problems that were present from working in his apartment to working in the office, than to the point where his group practice had over 5,000 sq. feet and 20 personnel. Work the time line and budget issues. Even though there is limited amount of information, this exercise can be studied from a number of angles: business, management, private practice, group practice, and forecasting of referral needs and future financial requirements.

CB&O

Personal Observations:

1. Visit a MHMR or Community Mental Health Community Center and ask how they handle infrastructure needs.
2. Visit a multi-specialty clinic and talk to the administrator about their use of infrastructure and what they consider more important than others.
3. Consider how some of the expertise listed in this chapter might be of help to your practice if you could afford them, on a time share basis or on a retainer or per hour or case basis.

References:

1. Frischmann, Brett M. <u>An Economic Theory of Infrastructure and Commons Management</u>, Minnesota Law Review, Vol. 89, pp. 917, Social Science Research Network, <u>www.papers.ssrn.com/sol3/papers.cfm?abstract id=704463</u>, assessed 5/01/06.

2. The Illinois Chamber, <u>About the Infrastructure Council</u>, <u>www.ilchamber.org/ic/inf/h/infhome1.asp</u>, assessed 5/01/05.

3. Dixon, Jill, and Joan Buhrman, <u>America's Crumbling Infrastructure Eroding Quality of Life</u>, American Society of Civil Engineers, March 9, 2005, p.1, <u>www.asce.org/report/card/2005/page.cfm?id=108</u>

4. Chamberlain, Ken, National Mental Health Association, Newsletter, 12/2001, p. 1, <u>www.nmha.org/newsroom/bell</u>

Chapter Eight
Managing Chaos and Change

Summary

The practice of health care is a lot like being a shepherd over a flock of sheep. There is danger lurking around each rock, tree, or hill. The shepherd has to anticipate danger, monitor the work of his four-legged assistants who help him move the flock to greener pastures. For health care providers this includes managing constant interruptions and the ebb and flow of referrals; dealing with demands on one's energy, expertise and time, often without any help; understanding frequent managed care changes, new laws and regulations that can have a significant impact on the practice, and maintaining a constant guard against liabilities and other risks.

What you will learn in this chapter:

1. You will learn the how your practice can be bombarded with a host of unexpected changes.
2. You will learn how managerial techniques can be used to handle the flood of information.
3. You will learn how to manage programs and projects.
4. You will learn how to reduce the risks of liabilities.
5. You will learn how to handle fluctuations in the economic marketplace.

Managerial Skills

For many therapists it seems like that the longer we are in the business of therapy, the more we read about what we don't know, about what we ought to be doing, including what we should do, when and where we can do it and how long we must or can do it! While we feel like the shepherd to a flock of patients, we, in turn, often feel that the positions have switched with us and now we are the patient, now we are looking in, a member of the flock rather from the position of the shepherd.

Over the past 25 years there has been a significant use of surveys and polls which have incited fears of the unknown, and therefore, the numerous out-of-control feelings. We have searched for meaning in of the black forest of a more structured: continuing education courses. We have dived into the internet and an intranet with unlimited resources and information, with thousands of news web sites that offer e-mail updates daily or weekly. There has been an increase in cable and direct television services that have opened up dozens of news programs. It also appears that every week books, magazines or journal articles are being published that parallel and discuss changes in rules and regulations affecting our field of practice. With this flood of information pounding on our tiny practice beachhead, it is easy to understand how therapists feel regarding the erosion of their practices and of their abilities to practice.

In Texas we have lost up to two-thirds of the population we can service due to the current priorities of the budget-conscious legislature over the past two years. Therefore, if you have a significant percentage of Medicaid patients, you can no longer service adults with Medicaid, and a large percentage of former SCHIPS patients were not covered until the last month of the 2005. Those who have chosen to accept the challenge of working with individuals from the lower socio-economic levels of society find themselves seeing primarily children. If you happen to believe in working with schools and parents to gather history and progress reports, as well as to help shape treatment goals and plans, then you may be shocked to find that a growing number of schools are refusing to let their students out of school for any doctor appointment. And some are refusing to allow therapists to see students in the school. Therefore, the hours one can see children are from 3:30 to 8 p.m. or on Saturdays mornings. These restrictions underline the therapists' need for greater controls of time and resources.

It means cutting debt, finding ways to accept more Employee Assistance Program (EAP) patients as well as expanding third party exposure to fill vacant scheduling times during the day. The problem with EAPs is that they can pay $30 an hour. That means you take a lost every time you see a case. That's almost 60% less then what Medicaid pays! The only way you can make higher is to re-negotiate with the company who has the EAP contract or get the contract for yourself.

These strategic decisions and actions are within management purview. Practitioners have to make decisions about the times they can patients, what type of patients they want to see, where they will see them, if they will accept a sliding scale (another reduced payment), and what panels they need to be on. The practitioner has to determine how many lower-than-Medicaid payments he or she will accept, and no vendor is going to reduce his or her rate, the lease isn't going down, and the phone company won't accept a sliding scale. Therefore the therapist, as a practitioner-manager, has to make business decisions. He or she may turn away patients, even though those patients are needed to fill up the day. Turning patients away may seem counter productive, but it can also save slots for higher-reimbursement-rate patients who can reimburse the practice at a rate that is 3 or 4 times than what might be offered for a person without insurance coverage and no steady job.

Therapists may not "feel" like they are managers, and few would describe themselves that way. Most definitions define management by describing techniques. For example, management has been defined as the "coordination of human and material resources to award objective accomplishment" (1) The following are some examples of management actions. You could be a manager if you do the following:

- make any plans (patient, scheduling, work schedule, things to do);
- perform case management;
- prioritize (callbacks, office chores, office policies and procedures);
- assign any duties to subordinates;
- organize your computer, files, billing;
- have ownership for the bottom line and spend time with your accountant or certified public accountant preparing monthly or quarterly balance sheets for the bank and for tax returns;
- develop some type of marketing plan, brochures and other advertising material (business cards, newspaper ads), attend seminars or community meetings for networking exposure).

Information and Data

In reality, psychotherapists have been exercising managerial muscle without seeing these techniques as management techniques. For example, good listening skills are important in a good manager. Taking adequate notes (progress, or for the files) is also something that effective managers do. If the psychotherapist gathers information from relevant sources for collaboration or clarification it can help in developing a treatment plan and monitoring the success of the treatment plan. The same is true for management. Managers need to know how and where to collect relevant, adequate and accurate information before making decisions. When psychotherapists collaborate or consult they are gathering information about how their patient responds to re-directions, confrontations, discipline, and anger or frustration. They are checking how appropriately the patient responds to important peers and authorities (adults) in his or her life. Managers can use a communication audit to determine the effectiveness of communication within the workstations, departments and the entire organization. They can also survey the effectiveness of vendors, or other sources outside of the building (i.e., headquarters in a different state) or the community local area network (LAN) system. Behavioral modification (therapists) is similar to management by objectives (managers). Both have stated and written expectations of behavior and the consequences attached to the behavior (positive, negative, or ignoring).

Managing information is important to a practice because information helps with forecasting expenses, can increase the effectiveness of a practice, can decrease professional liability and one's liability under state and federal regulations and can provide timely information about new techniques for disorders one may be working with, and can help with balancing a budget. The best information is the type that arrives in a timely fashion; is accurate, adequate, understandable and relevant; and is in an accessible form (fax, e-mail, and regular mail).

An excellent way to save and retrieve information is to use a database. Databases are written for different purposes. It's important to hire an expert to help develop your database, or to advice on the software program that fits your practice. Information and databases are both assets and liabilities. As the years fly by the number of patients you treat, the number of families you assist in some way, the categories of treatment you administer, the treatment plans that worked or not, and the demographics of those you treat are examples of information that can be extremely beneficial in audits and forecasting. The names and addresses can be used for sending satisfaction questionnaires, something auditors love to see. Information is also an asset for developing a marketing strategy. From the data base you can choose different sets of logistics to aim the ad to such as families with young children exhibiting oppositional behavior. While a database may be an expensive initial investment, you may find that it is <u>more expensive</u> if the information is NOT consolidated in a database

A database is useful in the accumulation of patient data for statistical review, auditing, cost analysis, and forecasting. A database entry is made for every activity on a patient. All mental health codes (DSM 4) and medical services and procedures codes (CPT) are entered on each chart and entered into the computer system by the database technician. There are several types of database software, but for a small group practice, many agencies create their own, often with the help of a computer consultant.

A database can help organize many different types of information, such as:

- types of services and programs provided
- frequency of services
- patients' ages
- patients' ethnicities
- patients' educational backgrounds
- schools and school districts served
- nursing homes served
- insurance payers
- how fees were paid (insurance, sliding scale
- private pay (if different from sliding scale)
- free services
- therapists providing services
- patients' birthdays (sending out monthly birthday cards is often

a very small but appreciated service)
- geographic locations of patients
- referral sources

Services

Health care is a service industry. It's not selling a product like cars, furniture, or fax machines. Services are intangible. When a psychotherapy service is purchased the patient is buying a performance provided by the seller. After a few days the purchaser may have to return for more of this service to meet their daily life needs. This intangibility makes advertising and promoting a service-based business more difficult. Marketers have found that the best way to sell a service is to focus on the provider rather than the product.

"The service provider usually has a level of skill and expertise that represents the service. As a result, advertising often focuses on the skill and technical competence of the service provider... It is important to ensure that the service provider is presented as a credible and knowledgeable source of service." (2) In rural and border communities it is also important to emphasis "staying power." In other words, it has to be clear that the service provider is established in the community, and/or that the service provider will be serving the community for years to come. For example, sometimes patients don't go to a new doctor until he or she has been in the community for several years.

There is a down side to the service industry. If the provider has a "bad" day the patient may not come back. If the provider suggests a procedure the patient doesn't want, the patient may not return. If the psychotherapists confront destructive behaviors or irrational thoughts, the patient may choose to hold onto those behaviors and thoughts and move on to another therapist who won't confront the patient. My German friend, Jurgen Kohler, is a small town banker who stresses the value of service and how banks and other businesses compete for customers by providing more personal contact and services people want and need. He lives in Eltmann, Germany, and spends time talking to local citizens who bank at his bank. Just talking with them, having lunch, providing the attention most people value, like listening to their needs, is something that hasn't lost its place in a busy marketplace, even in a small German community. If it works there, why wouldn't it work in your community?

Working In A Changing Marketplace

One of the most influential economic theorists, Adam Smith, wrote the landmark book, *An Inquiry into the Nature and Causes of the Wealth of Nations,* in 1776. His theory was tabbed "laissez-faire" because of his concept of the "invisible hand" in the marketplace which affected the outcome of the distribution of wealth. He theorized that if the government stood by and just let the market work without any interference, it would grow and everyone would prosper according to his or her efforts. His theory argued that competition would be the control factor in the marketplace. While that may be true in part, there are other control factors in the marketplace that affects the costs and value of health care services.

Such factors include policy makers from different disciplines outside of health care such as politics, the judicial, educational and the business field. In 1858 Charles Darwin's *Origin of the Species* was published. He argued that within the biological organism the strongest could be expected to survive. In the marketplace, too, the rich and powerful ones dominate. This is evident in the health care field, where HMOs, MCOs and large hospital organizations dominate the marketplace. They dictate, intimidate, and outspend health care providers. They are the movers and shakers standing tall above the professional associations and health care groups. They influence the legislators and train and influence the staffs who write the health care laws. The states have given these mega- bucks organizations a field to play in, and practitioners who work in those fields must play by the rules that have been established by the giants.

According to Tuckfelt, Fink and Warren (Managed Care in the 21ˢᵗ Century, 1997, we have the opportunity to run or fight. "There are two types of psychotherapists in this category: those who have problems getting on – or remaining on – the lists of MCOs, and those who choose to work outside of managed care for personal reasons. Psychotherapists in either or these positions might consider a specialty that is needed by people who are willing to pay for their own treatment." (3)

During the Great Depression economist John Maynard Keynes' book, *The General Theory of Employment, Interest, and Money*, (1936) was released. His basic theory was that by consuming we can save money and resources because consumption is the best way to reach full utilization of resources. According to his theory the government is the external force that provides the balance necessary to ensure full employment so that people would have financial resources to consume. Politicians have run campaigns on the idea that by cutting taxes we can increase revenue. This economic theory suggests that if people have more money in their pockets they will spend it. When they buy something they contribute to the growth of the economy. More sales, more jobs, more people buying more widgets.

Today politicians are faced with red ink on their budget books. They can raise taxes and collect the revenues they need, but they fear that voters will vote them out of office. There is also the concern if the taxes go up people will have less to spend, and that could lead to fewer sales, higher unemployment, and even less tax revenue. Governments need higher employment for several reasons so that more voters are working, more people are earning money to spend, and employers are paying for the health care of more people.

While governors are spending millions of dollars to attract new businesses to their states, they are taking those millions away from social service programs like health care for the poor. Government needs high employment rates (not full, but high) in order to have employers who can pay for health care. However, even with a low unemployment rate nation wide, there is debate about the high cost of health care. State governments have cut off hundreds of thousands of children and low-income families, and they have decreased reimbursement rates to providers. HMOs and MCOs have followed with their own increased restrictions and reduced reimbursement rates. Medicaid has sold out cases for case manager Medicaid cases to MCOs. More money is going into these MCOs and less into the pockets of providers. No wonder physicians as well as non-physician providers are pulling out of panels or not signing up when another MCO comes to town, as they seem to do every 18 months or so. While there appears to be some sign that the MCOs and HMOs are seeing shortages of providers, these shortages have mainly been among nurses, primary care physicians, and some specialists. So far the MCOs and HMOs feel that there is an abundance of mental health providers, social workers, and chiropractors.

These discussions are forcing more and more coffee house conversations about trade-offs. Do we want to pay for a $20,000 surgery or for a new school building? Do we want to pay for every child and one out of four adults to have health care, or do we want to limit who is eligible for Medicaid coverage? Who makes these choices? Right now government and their HMO and MCO comrades are in the decision-making position. Recently people have successfully sued HMOs for not authorizing payments for procedures. In a more than a few cases people have died because their doctors couldn't get authorization for payment.

Therefore, some people have been able to penetrate the MCO fortresses to gain coverage after being denied.

David Cutler, who served on Hillary Clinton's Health Care Committee during the '90s, has proposed a different way of addressing health care financing. He believes we need to address the values medical care can provide. Second, we need to pay more for quality care. He writes this while state governments are cutting services and access due to lost revenues. Employers are cutting back on coverage and increasing deductibles and co-payments. Philanthropic foundations are having problems maintaining funding levels. Now David Cutler suggests that it's not the money that is the problem, it's the value. "The goal of medical care is to improve our health. The system works well if it improves health sufficiently to justify its cost, and poorly if it does not. That seems obvious, but it has deep implications. Most significantly, it implies that controlling medical costs is not an important goal in itself. Lowering costs is good if we are overspending, but bad if we are getting valuable care. We need to ask whether we are getting enough for our money, or whether the money we put into medical care would be better used on food, shelter, or other items." (4)

As this dialogue continues it is important to continue searching for more information. New articles are coming out each week on the Internet. Newspapers are covering these issues in editorials and many times on the front page. It should be obvious that to make quality decisions, not just selfish and narrow decisions, we need more information. While this holds true for the issue of health care, there are the on-going issues of HIPPA and confidentiality and the increasing costs of staying in business.

Ongoing enterprises contribute significantly to the body of knowledge comprising organizational theory. "We need continued observation and conceptualization from astute practicing managers.

Meanwhile, scientist-scholars have become more and more involved in research related to organizations but carried on in the context of basic disciplines. Those who engage in the work of basic disciplines have become increasingly aware of the pervasiveness of organizations in society and have begun to concentrate attention on relevant problems." (5) Industrial and organizational psychology and sociology are prime examples. You will find management techniques and theories have a lot in common with "real life" experiences. There are numerous books on how psychology and business blend together to define, to shape, to explain, and to control factors that affect the bottom line.

Costs

What is the bottom line of psychotherapy? A net satisfaction? Net profit? Best practice development and its success, in large part, depends on <u>our</u> integrity to <u>our</u> goals, the strength of <u>our</u> commitment to <u>our</u> goals, how we manage <u>our</u> time, costs, and information, and how and how quickly we react to changes. If we are confined to 5 or 6 hours of sessions per day, will we have to work Saturdays to pay our overhead? A Medicaid reimbursement of $52 per hour times 6 billable hours per day equal $1560 per week unless you work Saturdays. If you could repeat that number every week of the month, that would translate in to $6240 per month. If you add Saturdays, at the same rate, that would increase your monthly income by $1200 for a total of $7440. Most practices have a 20-30%no-show rate, which is even higher for Saturdays. A 30% no-show rate 6 days a week for 4 weeks amounts to $2232 in lost income. That brings the projected total of $7440 down to $5208 and change. Then you pay the rent, the phone bill, and the answering service. You cover the costs of a computer, printer, fax machine, and paper and supplies. Add to that your other operating expenses, your taxes, and your accounting and legal expenses. Even if you do your own billing, do the payroll yourself, and personally take care of accounts payable, your monthly net gross income will be in the neighborhood of $2000. If you did this for 12 months that would add up to a net income of $24,000 a year. With rent, food, entertainment, retirement, car payment, plus car maintenance and the price of gas, are you willing to work for $25,000 for one, two or five years before you are able to join a group, increase your referrals or/and hire contract therapists to help you? How long can you work without a vacation, without taking off holidays, or without taking sick or personal days? Managing your time means managing the known expenses as well as the unknown or unexpected, especially when you don't have much margin with which to work.

If we have to work without taking days off, or if you have to work a 6-7 day week, how long can you be effective? There will be weeks (Spring Break, Thanksgiving, Christmas and Teaching and Knowledge Skills Tests {TAKS} other testing weeks) when school children will not or cannot be seen. Then there are the summer months when they leave town for vacation or they are children of migrants who leave in April and return at the end of October after working up north, or the parents "forget" their appointments or have something else they want to do.

In the end, if you have a solo practice or a group practice of any size, you are an entrepreneur. An entrepreneur is a businessperson. A businessperson is a manager. Learning the techniques for effective management can help you understand your role and suggest ways to improve your bottom line. To be successful you need the same information as the "big boys" have. You may have to settle for less equipment because you can not afford the additional labor costs. You may be able to gain the information you need from the internet. You may not be able to hire people to fill the professional infrastructure needs, so you can either do it yourself or outsource it or hire consultants.

One other opinion may lead to joining a group practice as a partner or full or part-time employee.

The business of psychotherapy is like a kite that depends on us to get it off the ground, and guide it though the clouds of uncertainty. We must know when to bring it in from the storms without crashing into bankruptcy or legal demise. The owner has the controls but needs information, and perhaps a little luck, keep the kite flying high so that it survives the harsh winds of change and practice interference by government regulators and HMOs auditors and contracts.

Marketing Strategies

Marketing is seldom talked about in medical, psychology, mental health, or social work graduate courses. Most business schools offer some type of marketing course in their undergraduate programs. Most hospitals hire marketing representatives who call on physicians, therapists, and social workers and encourage them to send patients to their hospitals when it is medically appropriate. Many of these "marketers" have little graduate training in marketing and business, while others have not even had a course in marketing in their undergraduate programs. There may even be a few who did not go to college. Unlike the non-health-care businesses, the medical field has not always been aware of the skills needed as a "marketing" representative. It takes more than a few lunches to attract some providers. Getting a free lunch is nice; having a pleasant conversation outside of the office is very nice. But building the relationship is harder and takes more attention to detail. For example, hospitals asking for referrals are sending these referrals through the emergency room. When a mental health patient goes through an ER, there are numerous ways to get lost. Many ER personnel have little knowledge of, experience with, or even motivation to tackle mental health issues. Opening a own private practices without any marketing and business courses is like opening a grocery store because you like to eat or because you like to shop. Passion for a field does not make you successful; knowledge does. Marketing involves knowledge because you have to know how to identify and satisfy customer needs and wants. Effective marketing requires you to understand how your clients make decision, how their habits will affect their interactions with you, and how their needs affect their decision.

For instance, since the young generation probably eats more candy then those living in a retirement center you might want to consider setting up a store that sells candy in a family community. If you are opening a convenience store look what other c-stores are in the area you want to reach. And since it most c-stores sell gasoline you may want to select an intersection and if you are near a major freeway that might be a better location then in a bedroom community. Would you be willing to invest $50,000 so you could rent a store to wait for people to come in and purchase your merchandise or do you want to go out and find them (in store selling or internet/newspaper ads/door-to-door leaflet)? If you are going to open a clinic or office you need to do your homework about the population that is in the area you want to work. Plan you strategy by the services or products you want to sell and then study the population and then the best location.

Those choosing to start a private practice will be looking to establish a position in the community or neighborhood that would make you "superior" in type of services or quality of services or quantity of services or makes you easier to reach. Or you might want to sell your services as less expensive. This is called making a "niche" in the marketplace. A "specialty" is the decision to offer only psychological evaluation services or drug and alcohol counseling. A "niche" has two elements:

> (1) a narrowly defined group of individuals to whom you target your services; and

(2) a "program" that you can sell consistently to one group or modify to reach out to new markets. A market niche refers to the population your service or product that is aimed at for consumption or use.

First, you could serve a specialized market by offering mental health services to a geriatric population in nursing homes. Second, you could develop a geographic niche by restricting these services to a geriatric population that only live in nursing homes in one country in your area. Third, you could offer a narrowly focused service, mental health assessments, to this population. Fourth, you could offer mental health assessments only to in this population whose insurance carrier is Medicaid. You could specialize even further by offering mental health assessments only to terminally ill patients within the selected population.

If your chosen market niche is too large and lucrative, it might invite competition. If it is too narrow, you could starve. Finally, if left undefined, you could get lost "in the crowd." Opportunities in the marketplace are constantly changing. A therapist, psychologist or physician will do well to be aware of these changes and how they affect his or her practice and services. Some of these marketplace changes could include the following:

- the increasing proportion of working women;
- changes in purchasing roles within the family, i.e., women with children with behavioral problems are bringing their children into therapy, whereas men tend to "suck it up" or "keep it in the family";
- changes in family composition;
- changes in the age composition of the market place, i.e., the increasing importance of the baby boom generation;
- the changing life styles and purchasing behavior of the women,

adolescents, men, minority individuals, etc.

- the changes in the population mix, i.e., in south Texas Hispanic people are in the majority; the impact of increasing migration due to immigration; and

- changes in technologies, i.e., the use of computers and telephones in therapies.

Cultural changes have had a profound effect on consumer purchasing behavior and corresponding marketing strategies. "Consumer values are standards of behavior that are shaped by society and important groups such as a family. Values such as achievement, prestige, social acceptance, and self-fulfillment provide marketers with guidelines in developing products and advertising themes. The 1980s and 1990s saw continued changes that began in the post-Vietnam and Watergate period, namely:

- "Me" orientation,

- A return to a "we" orientation,

- Greater emphasis on personal self-fulfillment,

- A trend toward a simpler life and reduced consumption referred to as 'Voluntary simplicity', and

- A skepticism of public institutions" (6)

Marketing is not just knowing the right location or being able to determine the needs of a certain population. It is complicated (there are multiple approaches or strategies), it is simple (telling someone about your services), it is vital (constantly changing), and it is an art (requiring constant revision). Marketing takes knowledge, experience, and time to develop. It is an on-going process that can be quantified.

Most practitioners cannot afford a marketing representative. If they can hire some one to help them with developing a marketing strategy and then working the plan, they will want to be part of the total program development and administration since no one knows one's business like the owner. Some marketing specialists call themselves "business developers." Business development is more than expanding or developing a practice. It includes strategic planning, public relations, network development, and, in small organizations, service on the compliance committee. Sometimes in a small group practice the business development director will work with the administrator and finance officer or CPA in developing a business plan for new programs, expansions, or buy-outs.

A marketing presentation is different than a clinical presentation in that it is more business oriented while the clinical presentation is more symptom oriented. Whereas a clinician will be concerned about feelings, a business approach is to focus on the bottom line. Whereas the clinician is concerned with taking adequate physical and mental histories, as well as histories of relationship development, academic achievements, and substance abuse histories, the businessperson is concerned with the history of the business and the success or failure of similar businesses in the community. Whereas the clinician is concerned with getting adequate health care providers and quality support staff, the businessperson is concerned with hiring adequately trained employees and a professional sales team. Whereas the clinician is concerned about state and federal health care laws and regulations, the businessperson is concerned with compliance with state and federal tax regulations that affect their industry. The clinician is concerned with therapeutic goals, whereas the businessperson is focused on sales or production goals. The clinician is concerned with behavioral and thinking change, whereas the businessperson is focused on the direction of his or her sales or production revenues. The clinician sees patients while the businessperson sees clients or customers. The clinician treats disorders. The businessperson makes or sells widgets or sells a service (doctor, chiropractor, social worker, family therapist, etc.).

As we learned in Chapter 2, the large corporation can have an advantage over a health care group and especially a solo practice or partnership. Deep financial pockets help large corporations protect themselves against allegations of fraud or racketeering, etc. They also allow these large organizations to have experienced and trained professionals to run keep departments like the Department of Human Resources, Director of Business Development, Vice-President of Sales, Program Project Developer, etc.

Every business operates within a marketplace that includes a diversity of businesses big and small, ethnic minority or majority. Not everyone frequents any one business all the time. There is even diversity among telephone companies and utility companies. If you sell widgets you may be competing against Wal-Mart. If you are a family therapist you are competing against every other counselor, social worker, licensed psychologist, or licensed family and marriage therapist. You may also be competing with a non-profit organization that may hire mostly non-licensed and non-degreed people.

The Effect Of The Economy On A Practice

The study of economics is the study of how to optimize the allocation of resources among users. Therapists are a resource for a community. Often therapists feel less a resource than a ping-pong ball. It's not a personal thing, rather it is a function of the marketplace and governmental agencies fighting to slam back costs and score points with the national economy.

In the marketplace there are conflicting interests and needs that are pushing therapists in different directions, sometimes at the same time. Employers across the nation are claiming that they are paying too much for health care. HMOs are raising their rates around 14%, blaming the hikes on all the claims they have to pay. Whole populations of people are underinsured or have no insurance at all. When they get too sick, they go to the nearest emergency room. ERs are filled almost 24/7 and are complaining they don't have the staff or resources to care for this population. Politicians are saying it's their priority to cut taxes and make the marketplace friendlier to the business world. Besides, they argue, it's not the government's job to be a charity organization. Adam Smith was a great supporter of a marketplace being left alone (laissez faire), believing that there are factors and resources in the marketplace that will balance it over a period of time. Governments run by dictators operate from the opposite theoretical orientation, using the government intervention to determine price, supply, vendors, etc.

An economy that uses both market and non-market signals to influence the allocation of goods and resources is called a mixed economy. Governmental influence puts additional requirements and boundaries on the practice of health care by cutting part of the playing field away. Instead of offering incentives, bonus, or higher reimbursement rates, they remind therapists that if they want to stay in the game they have to play by government policy makers' rules. Today, we see government central planning committees and agencies interfering more and more in the marketplace. These new policies makers may help the overall economy with their favorite economic policy, but they fail to appreciate the emotional and financial impact on a significant population. If these policies fail the social needs of society, it may take decades to return to a mostly marketplace-dominant playing field. Or the government may take over the whole game. In the meantime we may lose many of the best players and team members.

To balance state budgets, programs and services are cut or significantly reduced. Our political leaders may dash to their offices where they can slam home the message of "no new taxes." If they raise taxes the public will complain of having to give up shopping trips, eliminate vacations, or do without going out to eat. If the political leaders cut services, people lose jobs and businesses close. Employers look for ways to cut costs in order to handle the additional costs of lost contracts or patients. Employees or those on Medicaid lose money in that they must now pay more for health care. The uninsured or underinsured public can go to the ERs when they get really sick, or they can paddle across the border to Mexico or drive into Canada for cheaper medicine and medical services, or they may decide to choose alternative medicine or herbs, or find non-profit organizations for comfort and health care services, or they can just walk away from the table and do without.

Each state has counties without adequate health care (physical and mental). Conversely, each state has metropolitan areas that may have more than enough health care providers. This may be truer for mental health practitioners than for medical providers. The marketplace uses supply and demand to determine usage and price. When the supply is greater than the demand, the price is lower. When there is an overabundance of therapists, psychologists and social workers in a community the price of services will tend to be lower. HMOs use these numbers to set reimbursement rates. Central political and governmental budget planners do the same. This partly explains why Medicare and Medicaid reimbursement rates are so low. There has been an over abundance of mental health care providers for at least six years in metropolitan communities. If the politicians can cut $5,000,000 from the state budget they will do it, even though it means effectively taking away psychotherapy and other services. According to the Robert Wood Johnson Foundation, "Texas has the highest rate of uninsured working adults at 27 percent." (7)

Political agendas influence how funds are distributed across state programs. Those with the most influence on the local politicians influence political agendas. These include lobbyists, wealthy contributors to campaign war chests, and very vocal constituents. Therapists, in general, have done little to add their voices to the influence peddlers. Many consider it unprofessional, others may view it as useless, and still others may decide that writing a few letters is all they can do. The American Medical Association (AMA), the National Association of Social Workers (NASW) and the American Psychology Association (APA) have had lobbyists for some time, and now a growing number of other associations are beginning to hire lobbyists to try to present the case for mental health issues to lawmakers. But none of the health care lobbyists compare to those representing the education, oil, automakers and insurance industries. Since we are the economy, we are part of the production and consumption of goods and services. The challenge that makes economics theory work is to keep doing better. This is done by creating more jobs and by providing better services for our communities. Reducing the incidence of poverty will also help. Giving people better health care and a chance at a higher quality of education. Designing and producing more of the goods and services that people want and deserve. (8)

The economy of therapy is the study of the sum of all of our individual production and consumption activities in the field of therapy. How we manage our private or group practice is based, in part, on the factors that are used in the production of other goods and services (land, labor, capital, and entrepreneurship).

Opportunity Costs

We have the **option** of accepting contracts or not. Many fear losing more patients and being knocked off panels if they refuse to accept a low reimbursement rate. Besides, another therapist will sign the contract and accept the lower fees. We have the **option** of cutting our practice hours in order to teach a course in an academic institution, or to write books, or to consult with local corporations. We have the **option** of becoming much more active with professional associations and supporting efforts to educate political leaders in the value of our services. We have the **option** to offer more community education and prevention presentations in order to educate the public of the value of our services.

These are called <u>opportunity costs</u> because every time we use our resources in a certain way, we don't use them in another way. The true economic cost is not necessarily measured in dollars and cents. It is measured in terms of some alternative activity. It is the flip side of scarcity. These costs are more relevant to individual decision making than they are to the state or national economy. It means taking resources from one place and putting them in another. If we don't like the French government's policies, we don't buy their products. If we don't want to accept low reimbursement rates, we don't sign those contracts or we attempt to negotiate an increase. <u>If we don't like being treated like ping-pong balls,</u> we can put our paddles down and walk away from the table, choosing other games to play and other ways to use our time and talents.

Risks

The practice of health care is the management of risks, a lot of them. These risks include clinical disorders, disease management, and practice liabilities. The moment we chose to accept a license we chose to accept the consequences of being licensed. If you have more than one license, a risk to one is a risk to all. Between the lines, around the corners, and in the shadows are lurking risks to our legal and financial position in the marketplace.

If you accept an insurance contract you accept certain standards of conduct and practice, and you accept the consequences of crossing the boundary. In many states, the state protective and regulatory agency is now demanding more information from therapists who treat children in foster care programs. This information includes the names of all the foster programs each therapist is contracted with and how many hours a week the therapist is seeing foster children from all foster home contracts. Most people feel this is proprietary information and not the business of foster program contractors or the state. The state comes back and claims that the contract states that all providers will comply with everything the agency requires, stated or unstated, written or implied. And it is the state that is forcing the foster care programs to collect this information. Failure to comply will mean that the foster program contractor will be forced, by the state, to remove all foster children from your agency and give them to another agency or practice.

Few people understand these intrusions and liabilities in health care practices. Last week we opened up the office and discovered that two MCOs had sold their Medicaid contracts to another company and that 35% of our cases were in jeopardy of being lost. No letters were received announcing that change. After several calls, including to the state insurance commissioner's office, we found the new MCO. We found the phone number of a senior vice president from their website and made a call. Two hours later we got a call from another high ranking officer of this MCO who is now expediting the paperwork to help us continue to see, and get paid for, the patients that were switched to the new MCO. What is really happening is that MCOs and HMOs are carving-up administrative dollars amongst several companies (sometimes within the same parent organization). As these organizations gain more financial clout they are using that leverage to demand more for less from health care providers. If you don't comply, you lose all the patients covered under their plans.

Clinical Cases That Can Increase Risks and Liabilities Include:
- family violence
- marital conflict
- child custody disputes
- patients with borderline personality disorder
- patients with narcissistic personality disorder
- patients with dissociative personality disorder
- patients with post-traumatic stress disorders,
- patients who were abused as children or those who are currently in an abusive situation, and
- suicidal or potentially violent patients.

Risk Management

We are not, however, without some options. One of these is the management of risks. In many circles the practice of managing risks and liabilities is call "risk management." To therapists this means identifying the risks and liabilities to the practice and then developing a risk management program, process, or set of procedures to defend the niche and the practice.

The term "defensive practicing" has been used to describe how physicians and therapists take into consideration any possible losses that might occur due to their prescription or advice before they write the prescription or give the advice. That may mean referring the patient for more lab work or for a second opinion. Or it may mean referring the patient for a psychological evaluation before suggesting medication therapy. Defensive practicing decreases the threat of losing your position on a panel, losing your license or being sued.

When you <u>screen patients for the severity of their disorders before accepting them</u> as patients, you are managing the risks of practice. When you refuse to accept Medicaid and Medicare patients you are reducing the threat of FBI involvement in an audit. Borderline personalities and suicidal patents are high risks. There are some patients who are both high risks as well as "high maintenance." Paranoid-schizophrenic and substance-abusing patients can be both high maintenance as well as high risk. However, while a case may be a high-risk case, it doesn't necessarily mean it is high maintenance.

Narrowing your patient load by defining and eliminating potential high risk and maintenance cases allows you to managing potential losses and risks. By <u>refusing to do home visits</u> because of the higher risks, liabilities and costs, you narrow the population you serve, meaning you will have to be more active in networking, marketing and advertising to attract more HMO and EAP business. Whether you are using defensive practice techniques or/and risk management techniques, today's therapists are forced by necessity to consider issues never discussed in any graduate course. If therapists have learned about these issues then they have learned about them from continuing education courses or journal articles or books. Best practice encompasses effective and exemplary techniques to increase access and quality of care. When you reduce threats to practice stability, you are influencing the risks and, hopefully, decreasing the chances for a complaint or lawsuit.

Risk Management techniques includes:

- Conform with all applicable legal and ethical standards
- In your practice's policies' and procedures' binder, write a compliance policy that includes the name and responsibilities of the compliance officer and compliance committee, to exclude the owner and include billing personnel.
- Include the notes from the compliance committee meetings in

the compliance binder.

- Hold the compliance meetings at least monthly..
- Earn continuing education credits and take courses on issues relating to ethics and the practice of therapy, including dealing with legal issues such as the HIPPA regulation.
- **Ask your attorney to draw up a compliance policy**. You may pay $2,000 to $3,000, but consider it insurance against allegations and investigations.
- Provide a way for employees to file suggestions or concerns that they do not want to offer verbally for whatever reason, i.e., a suggestion box.
- Purchase a professional liability policy that provides for legal expenses for a malpractice case and for an ethical violation allegation to your licensing board. The legal fees for representation at an ethics hearing for your licensing board can cost $2000 to $10,000.
- Have both regular internal and external audits of your practices.

Internal audits can be done twice a year with records of the audits noted in the compliance committee meetings notes. Recommend an outside auditor be hired by your attorney every other year to ensure compliance. Remember that Medicaid and HMOs will perform their own audits. Making the results of your audits available to them sets a good tone for your relationship.. Even if mistakes are found, in all likelihood fines may not be levied as long you as pay back any disputed "overpayment." An external auditor may charge $100 an hour but, again, its insurance and an investment against allegations and investigations. Also, ask your attorney to hire the external auditor in order to gain confidentiality and protect against the auditor turning your practice into an HMO or state investigating agency. These steps save you money in the long run.

- Document all terminations, including any referral sources given to a patient who was terminated for reasons other than that the goals of therapy had been reached.
- Refer all patients for medication evaluation where symptoms indicate medication as a best practice policy.
- Document all consultations.
- Include a suicide risk assessment in the progress notes for any patient with any suicidal or cutting thoughts and behaviors.
- Place all contracts for safety in the patient records (where the patient signs a statement that the patient won't commit suicide and if he/she has an impulse to do so, and that he/she will contact someone first.

Quality Assurance

Quality assurance (QA) is a form of risk management. QA programs attempt to ensure accountability as well as to prepare for audits, to provide valuable information to the compliance committee, and to provide proof of intent to comply with contracts and state and federal rules and regulations. State auditors examine the files for schemes and attempts to defraud the government. With the use of a compliance committee and internal and external audits, you can significantly reduce fines and penalties if, in fact, over-billing or a lack of adequate documentation or even a lack of a progress note(s) are discovered. If, during one of your audits, an over-billing is found, or a lack of progress notes is discovered, you should consult your attorney and your attorney will guide you in writing a letter of your findings to the insurance organization and making arrangements to repay the organization. Over-billings and a lack of progress notes happen.

People forget or are negligent. That doesn't have to mean that they are attempting to defraud an HMO, MCO or government. Proof of an attempt to comply with regulations and best practice concepts can usually reduce any allegation of "intent."

The Agency for Healthcare Research has developed <u>tools to assess the quality of mental health programs</u>. These tools can support your compliance program. Those agencies that contract with HMOs and Medicaid and Medicare can have their files audited for evidence of service planning, treatment objectives, patient input to the process and consultation with the Primary Care Provider (PCP) when appropriate.

Power Point

Change equals a certain cost. Chaos equals a certain cost. Lack of change equals a certain cost. Therefore health care providers need to be aware of the effect of change, chaos and risks in order to control costs. Without management of the factors discussed in this chapter no provider has much of a chance to survive in today's marketplace, let alone a profit.

End of Chapter Questions

Multiple Choice Questions:

1. Communication Audits is used to determine:
   a. Financial stability
   b. Communication effectiveness within an organization
   c. Communication effectiveness between organizations
   d. Effectiveness of MBO programs

2. A database is used for:
   a. Collection of information on files
   b. Collection of files for audits
   c. Accumulation of patient data for statistical review and forecasting
   d. Statistical data only

3. Service is a(n):
   a. Product
   b. Intangible
   c. Performance similar to entertainment
   d. Incalculable act for business purposes

4. MCOs are created to:
   a. Administer the delivery of an insurance program
   b. Build customer service centers
   c. Create networks
   d. Create insurance plans

5. David Cutler suggests that the problem with health care administration and delivery is the:
   a. The money
   b. The product or service
   c. The management
   d. The value

6. A marketing niche is the same as:
   a. Specialty
   b. Location
   c. A narrowly defined group and a program that meets their needs

        d. A major player on Wall Street

7. Assael described the changes that began in the post-Vietnam and Watergate period as:
        a. A greater emphasis on personal self-fulfillment
        b. A skepticism of public institutions
        c. A trend toward a simpler life and an increase in voluntary simplicity
        d. All the above

8. The study of economics is the study of how to:
        a. People operate in a vibrant marketplace
        b. Manipulate the marketplace
        c. Optimize the allocation of resources among users
        d. Build and manage an business enterprise

9. Health care providers work in a dangerous environment as a result of:
        a. Violence and abuse in families
        b. Increase complaints against providers
        c. The expansion of control and influence of MCOs and HMOs
        d. A and B
        e. All the above

10. Risk management techniques include:
        a. Write a compliance policy
        b. Purchase a surety bond
        c. Initiating regular internal and external audits of your practice
        d. Start a medical case management service as part of your services
        e. A and C
        f. B and D

Rethink:

1. Discuss how a service can have a down side.

2. How do QA programs attempt to ensure accountability as well as prepare for audits?

3. Go to the Internet and explore the tools of QA offered by the Agency for Healthcare Research.

4. How do you avoid chaos in an organization?

Personal Observations:

1. Discuss Information Technology, what it encompasses, how it is used in industry, and future trends, with an Information Manager.

2. Write a compliance policy.

References

1. Kast, F. and J. Rosenzweig, **Organization and** Management, McGraw-Hill, 4th Ed., New York, 1985, p. 7.

2. Assael, Henry, **Marketing Management, Strategy and Action**, Kent Publishing Company, 1985, p. 300.

3. Tuckfelt, Sondra, Jeri Fink and Muriel Prince Warren, **Managed Care in the 21st Century**, Jason Aronson, Inc., New Jersey, 1997.

4. Cutler, David M., **Your Money or Your Life,** Oxford University Press, 2004, p. xii.

5. Kast and Rosenzweig, p. 11

6. Assael, p.63

7. Houston Business Journal , May 12, 2004, p. 1.www.houston. bizjournals.com/Houston/stories/2004/05/10/24.html

8. Schiller, Bradley R., **The Macro Economy Today**, 6th Edition, McGraw-Hill, New York, 1994, p.4

Chapter Nine
Future Weather Patterns and Other Wild Assumptions

Summary

To attempt to predict any trend or pattern of behavior or to forecast any aspect of the future is, at best, foolish. This chapter summarizes the issues in this book and points out some possible directions in which health care may drift over the next few years. These predictions might help you as you plan your practice and select location(s), population(s) and what insurances and alternative payment plans to accept. Additionally, this chapter will make several recommendations on how you can weather the storms of future winters.

In this chapter you will learn the following:

a. How fragmentation of health care services drive up the cost of services and no increase in quality of care.

b. The new models of health care delivery.

c. If health care is a "right."

d. How a conflict with value priorities adds to the failure of today's health care system.

e. Why reform movements have never succeeded.

f. Why there is a need for medical billers to have some type of certification and professional insurance or bonding.

g. How an ounce of prevention can help reduce health costs.

h. Why people are saying health care providers need more education.

i. Some lessons we can learn from the experience of Hurricane

Katrina that can apply to the health care crisis.

j.   Why the 30000-pound Gorilla is hanging around.

Fragmentation Of Health Care Services

It seems rather ironic that a year after President Bush's New Freedom Commission on Mental Heath, budget priorities changed and the funding was sucked out of health care programs in most states and used in other projects. Puff went all the hard work, now being reduced to ashes with all the other good intentions and promises from our leaders on Capital Hill. So much for the promises made to survivors of serious mental-health illnesses. Another slap in the face, another dose of snake oil medicine. The executive order called for programs and solutions for serious mental-health illnesses of adults and children. It called for a way for these members of our society to have the opportunity "to live, work, learn, and participate fully in their communities." (1)

Michael Hogan was the chair of the commission and was also serving as the director of the Ohio Department of Mental Health since 1991. The commission noted the fragmentation of the mental health infrastructure and the commission's desire to formulate strategies for improving the alignment of federal, state, and local policy and practice. The agenda of the commission, according to Dr. Hogan, "was focused on the goal of helping people to achieve significant and valued life outcomes as opposed to more narrow or proximate clinical goals." (2) Obstacles face patients including the stigma of being treated for a mental health problem, unfair limits and restrictions on insurance policies, and a fragmented service delivery system.

Three broad concepts emerged from the commission: "First, mental health and law enforcement and the courts, in local communities, should collaborate to engage people with mental illnesses who may have committed criminal acts, to divert them into appropriate supervised treatment rather than incarceration. The second notion is that if people did commit crimes and are tried, found guilty, and incarcerated, they are entitled to get constitutionally required levels of mental health care while incarcerated. The third emerging principle is that when these folks are released, linkages to mental health care are critically important." (3)

The Commission acknowledged the problems of integration and collaboration between agencies and services. The size of the different governmental agencies can be part of the problem, as well the fact that multiple levels of authority must participate in, sign off on, and support such inter- and intra-agency cooperation and collaboration. For example, the National Institute of Mental Health (NIMH) and the Substance Abuse and Mental Health Services Agency (SAMHS) and CMHS have never been able to really work effectively together to increase assess to quality and continuity of care.

For real collaboration to take place a new attitude needs to transform all governmental, political and professional organizations, and we may see the state take back control over these organizations. Judges tend to listen more to the streams that produce revenue in their counties. When county judges want to change the CMHS programs in their counties to do things like collaborate, the counties can face threats of the loss of the CMHS in their county if they do not become team players. It works for community centers those small communities where a university program obtains a grant to build the center and administer the over-all program using local people to manage and staff the centers. Public service programs are often bogged down by politics, turf domain, and nepotism. With the present budget cuts, medical infrastructure has basically been destroyed. The change of political parties is not likely to bring about instant change or add to the infrastructure so more people can access health care, including mental health care.

The answer to fragmentation is not incremental reforms. This piece-meal type of answer to a serious problem in our country today can not be pushed aside with a flippant response as incremental reform. Such an approach "perpetuates inequities both in funding health care and in the allocation of our health care resources. They limit choice of health care providers. None assures continuity of coverage and care. All incremental approaches substantially increase health care costs, and most current proposals assure neither financial security nor health security." (4)

New Models Of Health Care Delivery

CMHS Centers are funded by state grants and held accountable to both state agencies and county judges. The agencies have focused on serious mental health issues (bi-polar, schizophrenia, suicidal cases, mild to severe retardation) that are critical needs in most counties. To that extent they have been successful. On the downside they have failed to think as entrepreneurs and instead have acted more like bureaucrats; this has caused employees to show disdain for "consumers" who ask for services. It has also caused the agencies to withdraw from active collaboration with other community mental health agencies. Therefore, if there is to be a change in the way communities face the issues of **collaboration** within the different non-hospital health care services, a better agency to provide leadership may be the Area Council of Government Agencies, which could have an officer and staff that could respond to the Department of Health and Human Services. Such a department might be more effective in building coalitions in support of practice collaborations and handle initial issues of suspected health care fraud, as compared to the Attorney General's Office, which tends to be trigger happy when handling cases, even with skimpy evidence and inadequate information. But collaboration occurs frequently now, especially between primary care physicians and specialists like mental health, hospitals, and cardiologists.

Collaboration is more than just a word. In Seattle, Washington, a group of practitioners and several local health plans, health care organizations, and hospitals joined forces to address the lack of health care for a certain population in King County. Working together as the King County Health Action Plan, the partners have funded several programs, including the following: Children with Asthma, African-Americans with Diabetes, and Cancer Screening for Vietnamese Women. (5) Whereas collaboration is a matter of exchanging information in a timely manner between one or more providers, there is no structured organization in place to help fund the professional infrastructure needed to protect against ethical or criminal allegations and any risk to financial destruction. Such a structure is the **multispeciality** groups that are increasing across the nation but at a snail pace. "The challenge lies in the reengineering of the delivery system, as stipulated by the Institute of Medicine's (IOM) <u>Crossing the Quality Chasm</u>. Its detailed description of key delivery system characteristics can be seen as a virtual blueprint for expansion of the multispeciality group practice model. The report envisions a delivery system capable of meeting six changes: (1) evidence-based care processes; (2) effective use of information technology (IT); (3) knowledge and skills management; (4) development of effective teams; (5) coordination of care across patient conditions, services, and outcome measurement for continuous quality improvement and accountability." (6).

As **CMHS agencies become more of a contracting organization** then a provider of mental health services we may see more internal conflict in communities between the county and professional medical and mental health organizations as well as complaints from those in private practice or in small groups who will likely be the biggest losers. It is already very difficult to practice without infrastructure of personnel, services and financial resources. It will get even more difficult as larger multispeciality groups swallow-up referrals and contracts from a more regional controlling organization as the county or university run CMCSs.

An **integrated community-based approach**, coupled with an understanding of the social roots of disease, is essential if equity in health is to become a reality for America's poor. People want the best health care they can get without paying more than they make in a week or losing their homes in bankruptcy. Providers want to make a living doing what they like to do, but they don't want to have to keep making calls for issues of coverage and pre-authorizations and they don't want to practice as if the Attorney General is in the room with them. A community-based practice model may be a way to reach all these goals. For example, a number of physicians, mental health practitioners, chiropractors, nurses, etc., willingly join a multi-specialty group in order to pool resources for defensive purposes as well as to have adequate infrastructure to offer adequate health care to patients. Otherwise they cannot bill for some policies, such as Medicaid and Medicare.

Health care teams are a growing trend. Usually the teams are composed of practitioners from a variety of disciplines who work together to solve health care problems. The growth of health care teams has largely been spurred on by the increasing number of patients over age 65. "Fifty percent have at least one chronic illness, and within this group, about three-fourths have more than one chronic illness. Caring for these individuals with multiple chronic illnesses requires the expertise of many different individuals in a variety of disciplines. In fact, it takes teamwork and an ongoing exchange of information. Patients themselves are important members of these health care teams." (7)

According to Dr. Shortell the ultimate goal is to have activated patients interact with these teams. There are three dimensions that are particularly critical in the use of the Chronic Care Model (developed by Edward Wagner) in treating any chronic care disease/disorder:

(1) adequate decision support, which includes systems that encourage providers to use evidence-based protocols

(2) delivery system redesign, such as using group visits and same-day appointments

(3) use of clinical information systems, such as disease registries, that allow providers to exchange information and follow patients over time. (8)

Another new model for health care delivery is the **cross-sector partnerships** in health care. Over the past 20 years there has been a movement of two giant entities heading for a collision. "The first is health consumerism, moving from emancipation, to empowerment, and on to active engagement. Coincident with this has been the explosion of the Internet, disregarding boundaries of geography, class, religion, race, and politics, and carrying empowering health language and knowledge to a global population increasingly at risk for the health decisions of themselves and their families." (9)

These two forces are demanding progress in health care delivery, administration, financing, the diminishing of inequities between mental health and physical health insurance polices, end of disparities of health care accessibility between rich and poor populations, and less tolerance with health disasters such as HIV or SARS. "Beyond the desire for collaboration, there must be environment readiness to ensure success. Desire to truly collaborate is reflected in the various sector's willingness to mutually plan, to align goals and objectives, to share risk, and to exhibit a good understanding of each other's strengths, weaknesses, and capabilities. True readiness is evidenced by an appreciation that healthcare is a local phenomenon reflected in concrete and realistic planning, and the design and management of the realities of time, place, people, institutions and target geography." (10)

Another model is the **free-standing clinics or practices** that concentrate on a large cash-only population. Medical doctors are charging a retainer (i.e., $10,000 for a family of four) in exchange for a promise that the doctor will be responsive the family's needs 24 hours a day, 7 days a week. Then the physician bills the insurance company for each service provided. Others only accept cash, but offer to provide information and billing codes to patients who wish to bill their insurance companies themselves. Physicians, chiropractors, mental health social workers, and therapists have begun to refuse Medicaid and Medicare, or any third-party insurance policy or MCO. Some physicians have cut their services and are now only offering second opinions and consultations. There are those people who are looking for an answer to their fears and anxieties who do not wish to have their insurance company to know that they are receiving mental health services or some medical procedure. While many of these practices take several years to develop, they often find that fewer restrictions allow for lower overhead and more time to pursue other interests. They also report relief from the fear of having a number of organizations that may wish to tell them how to practice their trade.

Some might argue that the root cause of health care problems today is in the way providers have competed for patients. Providers as well as hospitals and MCOs and HMOs have acted as if health care services are a commodity, a widget that can be manipulated to bring the highest price while created at the lost cost. Thus producing a higher margin of profit. The only ones who have profited have been the middle men and women who work for the MCOs and HMOs. They have the power to manipulate health care access more than the providers. They have used lower reimbursement rates, redefining what is of "medical necessity" and restricting access. We can expect these organizations gaining more power and financial positions within health care in order to be in position to profit from a national health care program.

As different models of health care are created, the issue of patient no-shows and frequent re-scheduling needs to be addressed. This problem, people not showing up for an appointment or calling in the day of the appointment to re-schedule, causes an increase in health care costs and current patients do not appreciate the problems it creates for providers. While some MCOs and HMOs may allow for a $25 fee for not cancelling prior to 24 hours of the appointment, Medicaid and Medicare programs do not. This encourages providers to get creative with such patients like multi-bookings at the same time frame or refusal to re-schedule or see the patient again, and a cut-back or refusal to see any more patients with Medicaid and Medicare policies.

Health care is a business and as a business the industry is susceptible to fluctuations in the market place (i.e. increased expenses without ability to increase premiums or costs per service), daily anomalies (i.e., no shows), and competition (i.e. alternatives to your services). Although many providers do not use the "c" word, competition is a daily affair. Not only is there competition from other health care providers with your specialty, there are other sources of pain remedy or alternatives of your services. There are a number of people that urge more competition in the practice of health care. "Competition is a widely recommended cure for such ills (soaring costs, quality deficits, and growing numbers of uninsured people), but there is disagreement over the appropriate nature of competition: Should it be among integrated systems of care, as we have long advocated under the managed competition framework? Or should it be among individual providers and highly specialized groups, as advocated by some proponents of the 'consumer-directed', wide choice products that are gaining in popularity?" (11) The authors argue that competition among systems of care is the base way to encourage and stimulate high quality of health care.

Competition also comes from health care facilities outside the United States. We are familiar with the recent publicity of lower medication costs in Canada and Mexico. Less known, perhaps, is the high numbers of Americans that go to other countries for various treatments. Knee surgery can cost over $10,000 in the United States. In another country it can be around $1300 including the cost of travel. (12) Varicose vein surgery runs about $7,000 in the United States and about $1400 in another country including travel costs. Skin lesion excision is around $6300 here and $800 to include travel; Hysterectomy $5800 here, $2000 with travel in another country; and Cataract extraction is $3600 here, $1300 there. The savings can pay for rehabilitation-vacation in another country for several weeks! You can't get that here for those prices! Then comes the question of quality. A fair question when it comes to competition. One of the ways quality can be judged is through the eyes of the receivers. The largest study of U.S. health care quality suggests that all Americans -- rich, poor, black, white -- get roughly equal medical treatment from doctors and nurses and it is mediocre for all: Patients receive proper care only 55 percent of the time. This study shows that health care has equal-opportunity defects," said Dr. Donald Berwick, who runs the non-profit Institute for Healthcare Improvement in Cambridge, Mass.

"A well-functioning health care system should provide recommended levels of care 80 to 90 percent of the time, the study's authors said. Not only is no place safe, no one is safe from poor quality, Asch said. No matter what group we looked at, whether they were black, white, rich or poor, uninsured, insured, educated, uneducated, all of them were receiving mediocre care. He blamed the nation's fragmented and chaotic' health care system for making it difficult to deliver quality care. Greater use of computers could improve care by helping doctors track patients' medical histories, he said. In addition, computers could provide electronic reminders about needed tests and appointments. Electronic medical records could log information on other caregivers' thoughts about a patient's condition. Using 439 widely accepted criteria to evaluate the care they received for 30 common chronic and acute medical conditions, including hypertension, diabetes and heart disease, researchers found that it is almost a coin flip as to whether patients get the recommended care from doctors and nurses -- even though the standard treatments are widely known." (13)

Health Care As A Right

In some states it may be a crime for a doctor not to render aid at the scene of a car accident. But what about helping someone who falls to the ground coughing and clutching their arm or chest? Do we have a legal or moral obligation to render assistance? Most people in America would certainly jump in, irregardless if there is a Good Samaritan Law or not. There are plenty of stories of people reaching out and helping without asking for anything in return. I've been helped while stranded in the middle of nowhere, and I've tried to help others in similar situations. But if you own stock in a pharmaceutical company that sells medication at a price that most can not afford, are you denying people the assistance they need to live, or something that would at least decrease their pain and suffering? But is it a right by way of citizenship or "being in the country?"

Conflict With Values

People will ask why the system of health care is larger now than it was years ago. Historians may respond that in 1950 the medical system was very small. Secondly, economists report a comparison between yesterday's dollars and today's, for example, that health care dollars equaled $1 for every $25 spent in the marketplace in the 1950s. Today they report that its $1 for every $7, maybe $6. Some project that it won't be long before it reaches $1 in $3. For those of you who are old enough, think about what we spent for groceries in the 50s? For gasoline? Housing? It was much less then today. But when you compute it as a percentage of your income you may be surprised to find that the percentages are less then you think, except for gasoline, and if you live in California perhaps housing.

The issue isn't just about total costs, since there are more people living in the United States now then in 1950. The marketplace has exploded and the demand for housing, cars, clothing, food, utilities, education, entertainment, etc., has grown. Another issue is this: Are the prices of food, gasoline and housing going up, or are you getting more for your dollars? In health care, are spending more on individuals or are individuals using more health care? Finally, are we getting more for our dollars?

Many will argue that we spend more because we get more. In 1950 President Eisenhower was treated for a heart attack with bed rest, first in the hospital for 6 weeks and then at home for 6 months. Six weeks of bed rest at the hospital would cost a fortune today, and now there are other treatments that get the patient up and walking in a very short period of time. Vice-president Cheney is a good example. He has experienced heart problems that required surgeries that used to incapacitate an individual for six months. Mr. Cheney goes into the hospital and then goes back to work in a few days.

The treatment for depression has also changed. If you have seen the movie "One Flew Over the Cuckoo's Nest" of the 50s you saw how people were warehoused in mental institutions. Today they give those with depression Prozac or Zoloft or some other medication, but rarely are they hospitalized (unless it's for 3 or 4 days to stabilize a suicidal patient). Overall the costs of treatment have gone down. However, today we use medication and psychotherapy, and the number of people being treated has gone up. Therefore, the overall cost of treating depression in the United States has risen due to the greater number of people receiving treatment, not because the hourly rate has risen. The hourly rate for psychotherapy with a master's level professional was $20 in the 1960s. Today Medicaid's reimbursement is $52.51. That $20 from 1950 should at least $100 today.

We are making a mistake by just looking at the dollars per session. If you want to evaluate the benefits of mental health care you have to ask: Has the value gone up? To answer this question, consider these two benefits: morality and quality of life. While we are living longer, quality of life is much more difficult to measure. If saving a person from a suicidal gesture is saving a life, then what is the yearly value of that person's life if he or she lives another 40 years? What is that worth in the total scheme of health care dollars?

Since we are discussing the value of our health care dollars, consider that the costs of car air bags are $300 to $1500 depending on number of air bags and the make of car. I read once that the probability of you being in an accident and having an air bag save your life is about 1 in every 10,000 accident. That means airbags may run about $3-5 million per life. Per year that may average out to $125,000, depending, of course, the age of the accident victim and if they are prone to accidents. Since there is government support for air bags, then one can assume that $125,000 a year per person it saves from death is worth the cost.

If we are able to help a young first-grader get on medication, then train the youth how to handle his or her impulsivity, restlessness, and concentration problems, is the value calculated with a high school graduation, with graduation from business or nursing school, or when the person retires on a adequate pension and doesn't have to rely on Social Security? It is very difficult to measure the value of giving that child a better chance at a productive and less problematic life.

If we help a young mother get away from an abusive relationship, is the value of our work calculated with the life of the mother and child? It is the fact that they were able to access appropriate health care? Or maybe the value can be quantified by the fact that there was a therapist who accepted her insurance policy?

How do you calculate the value of psychotherapy and medications for posttraumatic stress disorder? Schizoid affective disorder? Panic attacks? Bi-polar disorder? Paranoid schizophrenia? We have yet to calculate these disorders in terms of economic value to the community. But we must! Because that is how the policy makers think, talk, and make decisions about our field of study.

When you read the polls, the first or second item of priority is health care. However, if you say, I'll give you a tax credit so you can buy more health insurance, do you think that most people will do just that? Or will they buy a car or another TV? We are having this type of debate now with social security when we discuss giving people money or credits so they can invest in stocks, bonds or mutual funds. Watch the comments from people on the street, from pollsters, and from politicians. What is the big fear? Perhaps politicians understand human nature and impulsive buying. They fear that people will return the tax credit to the marketplace without saving it. Americans tend to be lousy savers. They fear that people will refrain from using a health care tax credit for health care and will instead use the emergency rooms more, or will go bankrupt on medical bills.

Given the choice between health care and groceries, a majority of people may choose the short-term answer. The government's top advisors and policy writers will ask the same question. And they will get the same answer. The top advisors have worked in "think tanks," universities, and a variety of corporate organizations but they are not health care providers. They have experience with HMOs and PPOs, not one minute of experience in a rural community health center as a provider. The bottom line overrides any clinical symptom. They want more **bang** for THEIR dollar so they are more likely to look at the worth of our services to society. And where will they get this information? They can do some analysis on the physical medicine and physical therapy side, but the science and data of mental health counseling, family therapy, or social work is weak and may lack current economic value terms.

Policy makers and politicians at all levels of government argue that the budget has to be controlled or balanced. That means we do not spend beyond our budget allotment for any service or program. To do this several years ago many states cut all kinds of programs, including health care to the poor, even making accessibility to Medicaid and SCHIPS harder. According to some a more effective way to compete is to deliver the greatest value for patients. "Value-based competition will see more innovation as providers will not be all things to all people, but will create focused 'practice areas' that address specific disease and conditions with higher-quality, lower-cost services. Health plans will eliminate their restrictive networks, allowing members to choose in a competitive (and regional or even national) marketplace the providers that officer the best value for their condition. Plans will help patients make the best decisions by offering counseling and support services as well as information that assesses the relative value delivered by providers." (14)

There is conflict in leadership circles about the value and the "bang." While the leaders are insulated from the same financial and medical risks that most people are exposed to, the leaders have an unbalanced power over the general population in terms of determining the "values" of society and what quality and quantity of the "bang" they want to accept. The government decides that any amount is worth spending to fight this "mammoth" creature called fraud. So they build schools, such as the FBI Academy in Georgia, where they train agents and hire psychiatrists to attack health care providers. Psychiatrists are viewed as "public enemy number one" by many government law enforcement agents. They create technology to trap unsuspecting providers, such as the finger recognition machine that is being tested in Dallas. Patients are asked to provide a fingerprint the moment they arrive in an office and when they depart. The state claims it is used for weeding out "phantom" sessions/visits, but it is also a handy way to monitor and define psychotherapy or an office visit by minutes, not by what takes place during that time. This further emphasizes the quandary that law enforcement and politicians have. They don't understand what we do, so they assume we are defrauding the public with some form or "witchcraft" or scam.

The values-conflict, for health care providers, is that they aren't willing to see themselves as business people and entrepreneurs. This relates to the physicians who do not want to lose autonomy in their practice and resist joining a large multispecility group.

The first thing health care must do is change their point of view. **We need to understand, appreciate, and discuss the value of our work**. For clinicians the dominating priority is the health of the patient. The baseline of every organization is the coming together of resources to answer the questions: Why do we do what we do? At the end of each day have we performed duties and tasks that lead us to define our efforts in terms of success or failure? Have we reached our goals? Whether our goals are to pay our salaries, to make a certain profit margin, to see x number of patients; whether we have helped a family or made another widget or all the above. It's not all about money but it is not "not about money".   The entrepreneur, wither one is an owner of an auto parts store or a physical therapist, views his or her company in terms of ownership and ownership in terms of money. Investments of capital for personnel, equipment, real estate, or some other form of expansion are judged by bankers, accountants, and entrepreneurs in terms of the value of the dollar unit, and whether the investment yields a profit or not. All investments (start-ups or expansion) are made with the assumption that the investor (entrepreneur) is going to make a profit, assuming the marketplace continues to increase or remain stable and the business traffic to the company will also increase.

A second stumbling block to understanding value is the matter of eliminating waste. From the entrepreneur's perspective there is waste. Therapists and social workers and staff members who think they are working for the government tend to show-up, drink coffee, contribute to the rumor mill, and collect their checks. That may work in large organizations, but not is small companies. Although one would like to believe that all medical and mental health employees are devoted to their professions, it just isn't so. For some the passion isn't there. Their attitude is aggressive and turf-protective. They may be pleasant with patients but unreliable when it comes to doing all they can to increase the bottom-line. It's not their problem, it's yours. **They do not understand the value of therapy or medicine, and they certainly do not understand the value of provider time**. Every minute of every day there are costs accumulating: payroll costs, operating costs, fixed costs, variable costs, they all add up and must be accounted for; someone must be responsible for them. When a health care provider settles for less, the value of his or her services decreases and the costs go up for the company, for the patient, and for society.

A final value not often recognized but certainly debated, especially in utilization reviews or quality assurance programs, is the **value of performance**. We need to perform in order to heal broken lives. And we as a society need to value this performance and pay more appropriate reimbursement rates, perhaps giving bonuses or paying higher rates to those who can document greater effects from their services. And we need to find a way to reflect this value and these effects for society. Documentation leads to justification, which can have value for policy makers. Even without these values and performances adding to the quality of health care and reducing future expenditures, policymakers still need to be persuaded to listen and understand what we do, why we do it, and the value it has to society. The problem, however, still remains: the one with the deepest pockets calls the shots.

Reforming Alternatives

Since 1994, when the first health reform measures were initiated, not much has changed for the benefit of health care. In fact, things have gotten worse despite the growth of managed care. Today there are about 43 million Americans with no health insurance; 31 million Americans are underinsured, bankruptcies are up, employers are complaining about the rising costs of health care, and "health care costs as a percent of gross domestic product are projected to continue to increase, from 14 percent today, to 17 percent in 2007. The Health Insurance Portability and Accountability Act have not met the high expectations, demonstrating that the real issue denying easy solution is affordability of coverage. The Children's Health Insurance Program, while a step in the right direction, will leave millions of children uninsured. The burden of paying for health care continues to fall disproportionately on the poor and the sick." (15) According to the Consumers Union there are seven reasons for the failure of the present market-based health care system:

(1) Third-party insurance payment doesn't do enough to allow the consumer to be aware of the costs of health care;

(2) Americans tend to be too compassionate and do not favor letting people die who can not afford health care;

(3) Doctors are the decision makers, not the consumers;

(4) -Information is often slow, not adequate, not accurate;

(5) Employers choose health care plans, not employees;

(6) Costs of services vary from one provider or consumer to another;

(7) Special interests are dominant forces in shaping policy through their advocacy in Congress and with state legislators and insurance regulators. (16)

At issue is the crisis of health care funding. Over the past few years the stress has been placed on cutting programs but there have been others such as:

- Take money from one program to pay for another
- Using accounting tricks to mislead the public about the true deficit
- Borrow from financial institutions normally using bonds
- Sell-off assets, land, trees, buildings
- Invent a projection out of thin air, "Who would know the difference?"
- Cut employee benefits, cut use of heat or air conditioning or light bulbs
- Put-off maintenance and replacement projects to future years and hope for the best. (17)

Funding is at the center of most health care problems including reform suggestions. It starts with the loss of the traditional safety net that society has banked on over the years: Medicaid and Medicare. At the center of this problem are the converging elements of a "perfect storm". Such elements include:

- Higher health care costs
- Less money from the federal government
- A soft economy
- Increased drug expenses
- Fewer private-sector employers providing health care insurance
- An aging population with more medical conditions. (18)

When it comes to health care reform former House Speaker Newt Gingrich (R-GA) has stated that small cuts in budgets or Medicaid waivers here and there are not the answer. He favors legislation. Gingrich proposes establishing a program that would "provide incentives to people with disabilities to be productive, rather than threatening them with a loss of benefits if they can a get job; offering low-income residents vouchers for health savings accounts that educate them to the benefits of prevention, wellness, and early detection; and creating a program to reintegrate family back into elder care by allowing family members to financially contribute to beneficiaries' care without facing the risk of losing all Medicaid coverage." (19) Gingrich also claims that he is against a money-only program because he sees it as futile and a trap for the most vulnerable in society.

George Silver, professor emeritus of public health at the Yale University School of Medicine, argues that America's political leaders are clinging to the "dysfunctional health care system in the face of explosive evidence regarding the toll our choices have taken on our ability to protect citizens from the cost of illness and promote the well-being of our most vulnerable populations." (20) Silver goes on to suggest that approaches to providing health care have created a "supplier market like no other" where "industrial giants…have been enticed to the table by the promise of large profits and guarantees of total federal immunity from efforts to regulate their practices and businesses." According to

Silver, as quoted in the kaisernetwork.org newsletter, "Congress could take steps to restore the state capability for innovation and initiative through a program that appropriates funds and asks for a few basic things in return," such as a guarantee of service. (21) Hospitals are having a crunch of revenues and human resources, including nurses and pharmacists. For example, St. Michael Hospital, Milwaukee, Wisconsin and its parent company, Covenant Healthcare, are facing an $80 million loss over the past four years. Covenant, like others in the hospital business, is part of the effort to solve critical issues including the lack of primary care facilities and physicians, the inappropriate use of area emergency departments, and a gross under-funding of Medicaid. These problems face both providers and patients. "This is a social issue and it's a big problem," Covenant President and CEO Paul Del Uomo stated. "It costs hospitals $450 million just for Medicaid. This is not yet resolved. We are working on public policy issues that Covenant has taken a leadership role in. It's not a Covenant issue, it's a Milwaukee issue." (22)

According to *A Century Foundation Guide to the Issues* the following is a list of possible alternatives to the present way of doing business in health care.

1. Expanding Public Programs and Offering a Tax Credit. "This reform would merge existing public programs (Medicare, Medicaid, and the State Children's Health Insurance Program), expand their scope, and offer a tax credit for moderate-income Americans toward the purchase of health insurance."

2. Employer and Individual Mandates. "Building on existing employment-based insurance, this proposal would mandate employers to cover all employees and require employees to take this coverage. Premium subsidies would be offered to certain employers to enable them to afford the coverage they offer their

employees."

3. Individual Mandates with Tax Credits. "Under this model, the responsibility for obtaining health insurance would rest with individuals. Individuals and families would receive tax credits to help them purchase health insurance."

4. Single Payer. "In this scenario, the federal government would collect and disburse all payments for health care, set uniform benefit packages, create policies and standards for participation by providers and provider systems. Private insurance would be effectively eliminated."

5. Combination: "Eliminate the current tax breaks for employer-based coverage, consolidate government-run health insurance programs, to seek other sources of savings (such as gains, overtime, from improved public health), and then to use this re-directed money to subsidize individual and family-purchased coverage." (23)

Is there a climate for considering alternative financing for health care? A lot of people are talking about it, but that is where it has been for years and that is where it's at today. Unions, states, and corporate organizations have shown little willingness to pursue broad social alternatives. Unfortunately, the people and groups with a larger financial interest in the current system are the ones creating all the MCOs. "The elaboration of health care's corporate compromise not only drove health provision away from the state and into private bargaining, but also justified that choice by leaning heavily on the political, intellectual, and psychological framework of social insurance. Private bargaining, in turn, was shaped by the influence of race and gender both on labor markets and on the peculiarly American construction of social citizenship. Labor's notorious volunteerism underscored the ability of economic interests to turn the state against labor (and labor against the state), and the invocations to "manly independence" and "whiteness" woven through the history of American trade unionism." (24)

Certification and Malpractice Insurance for Medical Billers

While many practitioners employ professional medical billing services, there are still a lot who either do the billing themselves or have a staff clerk to do the billing. The problem is that too often billing clerks have only limited, if any, experience and do not fully understand the complexities of different HMOs and MCOs who have their own forms and pre-authorization procedures and requirements. Secondly, these "mom and pop" billers have nothing but their job at stake, whereas the licensed professional has his or her license and career at stake. Billing correctly speeds up reimbursements and reduces the number of memos needed to request more information or clarify or correct a policy identification number. At some point junior colleges will work with the state to build a certification for billers, which can also require some type of professional liability insurance or bonding to protect a practitioner from paying the price of an unscrupulous medical biller.

An Ounce Of Prevention

There are a growing number of groups who wish to see more preventive care in the United States. *The Wall Street Journal* reported that the nonprofit agency, Partnership for Prevention, "plans to launch a national effort to encourage adoption of strategies to promote prevention and wellness. Also, the U.S. Preventive Services Task Force intends to encourage providers to recommend preventive care to their patients. One recommendation calls for all patients to receive tests for 16 medical conditions, such as skin cancer, hip problems, iron disorders, peripheral artery disease, and genes linked with breast cancer." (25)

In addition to preventive care there can be another approach, such as advertising or marketing, to educated people about the effects of mental health on the physical body (present disorders or future illnesses or injuries), work stress, personal relationships, academic pressures, and on becoming more effective parents and grandparents. Americans have gotten used to ad campaigns to reduce smoking, heart attacks, strokes, and lung cancer, or to urge people to adopt more healthy diets and practice safe sex. But the use of such strategies for a psychological disorder, such as depression or suicide, represents a significant departure. "We have been missing opportunities to use public health promotion and prevention in the mental health sector," notes Alan Radke, who, as medical director for the adult mental health division of Hawaii's Department of Health, has been spearheading a broad review of prevention strategies for the National Association of State Mental Health Program Directors. "If we can demonstrate that the use of health promotion and prevention strategies works with suicide, from those learnings we can address any number of other conditions." (26)

The Competency Movement As A Bridge

Frequently we hear that there are too many medical errors and that people are dying due to the negligence of health care providers. These errors are said to cost the lives of thousands of Americans each year and to have left hundreds of thousands suffering chronic pain. "Education for the health professions is in need of a major overhaul. Clinical education simply has not kept pace with or been responsive enough to shifting patient demographics and desires, changing health system expectations, evolving practice requirements and staffing arrangements, new information, a focus on improving quality, or new technologies." (27) The Institute of Medicine report suggested the creation of a core set of competencies that could be incorporated into an ongoing educational program for health professions beginning in graduate school.

The reasoning centered around the mounting call of "society" for an error-free medical system, more accountability of providers, and demand from government agencies, MCOs, and HMOs for more quality control systems. They acknowledged that pushing providers to "try harder" doesn't work. They also acknowledged that working in the current system that does not adequately prepare them, either in graduate school or after they enter practice, and that doesn't offer them support (financial, educational, infrastructure), hinders the goals of a quality practice. The "system" they are attempting to reform is more of an educational system and has less to do with the administration and delivery of health care. They fail to include any acknowledgement of the business side of medical and therapy practice and they neglect the more pressing issue for providers, the exchange of values. In other words, how do we pay for all these changes? As providers are asked for more and more forms, procedures, and accountability there are additional costs that are not being acknowledged by these formable organizational bureaucrats. This is probably because none of them have had to earn a living as a provider. They have not had to be responsible for a budget or for marketing and networking to increase referrals and build up a practice. They have not had to manage an office staff to ensure that the business met its obligations. And when the revenues were not enough, they have not had to reach into their own pockets to pay the bills.

The Institute of Medicine IOM and its scholars are suggesting a plan that would have an impact on the curriculums of health care providers (medical, mental health, rehabilitation) as well as their programs of accreditation, certification, and licensure and would include "oversight" including **regional demonstration of learning centers**. These centers would serve as a form to check competencies throughout professionals' careers by periodically testing their ability to deliver patient care that reflects the oversight committee's list of competencies, among other requirements. If there ever was an example of Big Brother, this may be it. What makes it even more alarming is that the plan is being proposed by the IOM.

The Gorilla Will Continue To Hang Around The Neighborhood

At the beginning of the 20th century progressive reformers attempted to mandate health insurance for all industrial employees. The architects of Social Security considered national health insurance along with other social programs during the 1930s. New Deal reformers argued for it in 1949. Depressions and wars have also re-kindled this reform debate. In the early 1960's Congress debated a broad coverage of health care but settled for a welfare program instead. When Medicaid and Medicare were created in 1965 the reformers questioned if a more inclusive coverage might be more meaningful. Little by little the young gorilla in the closet has grown, fed by reformers' zeal and passion.

In 1973-1974 Senators Ted Kennedy and Wilbur Mills "retreated slightly on benefits, allowing private insurers to act as intermediaries, and relying on a combination of payroll-based contributions and taxation. The administration, reasoning that 'we can't beat them with nothing,' responded with a Comprehensive Health Insurance Program (CHIP) that combined a weak employer mandate with the HIAA's 1971 plan for subsidized private insurance." (28) Reform failed again when CHIP was perceived as trivial and worthless. One reason CHIP has been less then successful is that it pits employer mandates against cost controls and employers' interests against health care interests. Pitting one interest against another weakens both.

Health maintenance organizations (HMOs) were formed to control costs. It is suggested that they have only succeeded in filling their own pockets and have failed to control costs as expected. "Often the savings claimed by individual firms under managed care reflected not the ability of HMOs to deliver care more efficiently, but their ability to shuffle costs to workers and patients. Measured against past performance or the experience of other countries, the rapid growth of HMOs since the late 1970s has done little to check health care costs and has inflated the administrative costs of 'managing' and 'competing' that are largely responsible for the exceptional American cost crisis." (29)

Often health care reformers feel frustrated by the inability to convince political leaders of the value of health care for society as a whole. One of the reasons they have failed is that the corporate world contributes more to the pockets of politicians then do health care providers and other interested parties. Another reason is that corporate sponsorship is better organized. The AMA may be strong but they have refused to join with non-physicians because they have felt that such ties would weaken their voice with HMOs. Therefore, the healthcare providers have not been sharing resources or information and have not joined to create a larger and stronger force against corporate America. The third reason for not being very effective with politicians is that there are few if any health care providers who have run for office. Those that have were physicians. Fourth, the value of health care has not been described in terms that politicians and policy makers can understand and endorse. Finally, health care providers must be part of the think tanks and the policymakers in each state and in Washington, D.C. Today's reformers need to better document their work in economic terms, and in terms of value to American society.

Without having to reinvent the wheel, perhaps non-physicians can join forces with the labor movement and learn their techniques to promote ideas at the grass roots level. Joining forces with other professional organizations and labor unions can theoretically offer more political clout. Unfortunately, the labor movement has embarrassed itself by including unseemly characters in its organizational charts. They have lost influence, power, and membership because they have not been able to fight large corporations who offered more benefits and higher salaries then the unions offered. They also view "universal health programs as a threat to the referential tax treatment, and employer-financing enjoyed by job-based group insurance. By any measure, labor bet on the wrong horse. Employer provision has proved uneven and fickle, especially as deindustrialization eroded the actuarial logic of group insurance, and self-insurance, coinsurance, and managed care became the rule in the group plans that survived." (30)

"Just about everyone agrees that all people should have health insurance. The experience of the past decade teaches us that even a booming economy will not lead to increased insurance coverage without major public support," writes David M. Cutler. (31) What he offers is the program that already exists. The federal government offers several programs to nine million employees, including the president and members of Congress. The government organizes the proposed health care plans that will be presented to their employees, but it is private insurers that write the policies. Insurers must agree to accept EVERYONE and not to deny anyone.

For those who cannot afford to pay, subsidies might work since we have Medicaid now. Medicaid is financed through general taxation, the bulk of which is paid by middle to upper income individuals. Even hospitals offset their costs of care to the poor with funding from the county or/and state and federal government. To guarantee universal coverage, we need to compel people to buy insurance. This is a major step. In a voluntary insurance system like the current one, people have incentives to make the appropriate payments, or else they will not be covered. In a universal system, by contrast, people are guaranteed insurance, whether or not their check arrives on time. Universal coverage necessarily means a larger role for government than is the case now. "A consolidated insurance system of this kind – sometimes called a single-payer system – could eliminate many of the problems in today's hodgepodge of a system. However, sustained cost control and the realignment of incentives for physicians with the best interests of their patients will require still further reform in the organization of medical care. Fee-for-service private practice, as well as regulation of physician managed care businesses, will need to be largely replaced by a system in which multi-specialty not-for-profit groups of salaried physicians accept risk-free prepayment from the central insurer for the delivery of a denied benefit package of comprehensive care." (32)

The biggest difficulty in this or any universal coverage proposal is financing. Where does the government get the money to offset the cost of the tax credits? Put another way, the tax credits that the government can afford clearly depend on the available revenue. The foregone revenue from a comprehensive tax credit system is significant; a system like that proposed here might amount to about 5 percent of total federal spending.

With all the talk of reform, when will something be done? In other words a triggering mechanism. One view is that a political party will take it to the public during a presidential election and build up support for one type of reform. Another is that it will take a major catastrophe, a war, another national or world depression, or maybe a break-down of health care abilities due to flu pandemic that will blast a sudden change. We have experienced the destruction of New Orleans and the inabilities of civil authorities and agencies to prevent or respond quickly to the affects of disaster. The hospitals and nursing homes collapsed in more than one way. The Red Cross couldn't get enough mental health and medical volunteers. Most of the volunteers were "non-professionals" doing whatever they could to help other human beings. The federal government was in shock and detached at first and then responded but awkwardly. Pouring money into a project which was given birth by a disaster is only a temporary, piece-meal answer. As a country we can expect better. A pro-active rather than a re-active policy tends to be the answer that seems more logical. We can prepare for disaster or a disease or a disorder more effectively and efficiently than waiting for a flood, earthquake, or a diabetic condition to cause the lost of a leg or an aneurism to hit.

Obstacles Of Reform

There are a number of obstacles to reform. These include <u>those that are satisfied with the status quo</u>. A second obstacle is <u>attachment to one solution </u>without allowing for other options. The third obstacle is the <u>governmental bureaucracy</u> which can stall, change and lose any legislation without personal accountability. Those that gain from the benefits of the old way of doing things will fight to the end those who are the reformers. The fourth obstacle is <u>differences of opinion</u>, ranging from different perspective of the problems, differences in alternative approaches, differences in belief of who is "entitled", what services should be available to whom, and a basic difference in how resources are collected to pay for services and who is entitled to offer these services. A final obstacle is the <u>lack of a non-political organization of the administration and delivery</u> of health care. The current system devalues health care providers until there is an emergency or when politicians want to brag. "More than half of all physicians are in small practices; thus, they are poorly positioned to take advantage of advances such as information technology (IT), which could contribute to more efficient and effective care." (Victor R. Fuchs and Ezekiel J. Emanuel, Health Care Reform: Why? What? When? Health Affairs, Vol. 24, Number 6, November-December 2005, p.1401) Even more of the non-physicians are in private practice or small practices and can not afford infrastructure which would assist them in compliance and liabilities issues as discussed in earlier chapters.

No matter what plan we support, it won't matter unless you express your opinion to your elected officials. Become more active politically. Find ways to express your opinions. Get more active in your professional organizations. One start is to visit to the following website: www. practicenew.com. This website was created to keep you informed about legislation, new policies, and proposed legislation that can affect your practice or your agency, directly or indirectly, today and years from now. Getting informed, staying informed, and becoming a political activist for your profession and the values inherent therein, can be the difference in what direction public policy drifts.

Power Point

As long as managed care organizations are allowed to make huge profits and control both the providers and the patients, the demand for national health insurance will grow louder and more health care providers will find alternative revenue streams or even new jobs. Providers need to find new ways to get their ideas and feelings heard by policy makers and develop more effective ways to define and document the worth of their services to society.

⋐౩৪⋑

End of Chapter Questions

Multiple Choice Questions:

1. Over the next two years the government is expected to cut Medicaid benefits or reimbursement by:
   a. 25%
   b. 35%
   c. 50%
   d. 60%

2. What is essential if equity in health is to become a reality for America's poor:
   a. Passing and enforcing parity legislation.
   b. Integrated community-based approach, coupled with an understanding of the social roots of disease.
   c. Health care bonds that can be used to pay health care costs or premiums.
   d. A tax break that would be expected to use for health care costs.

3. What are keeping adequate physical and mental health care from all the people who need it?
   a. The lack of infrastructure
   b. The lack of will to build an infrastructure for health care.
   c. Not enough health care providers.
   d. Filters to accessibility.
   e. All the above.

4. Why do health care providers need more education?
   a. Lack information about the business side of therapy.
   b. To cut down on errors.
   c. Because clinical education simply has not kept pace with or been responsive enough to shifting patient demographics and desires, changing health system expectations, and a focus on improving quality.
   d. All the above.

5. The burden of paying for health care continues to fall

disproportionately on the:
a. Employers
b. Medicaid
c. Tax payers
d. Poor and the sick

Rethink

1. How has the current chaos in health care been affected by defragmentation?
2. Name three models of health care delivery that is being seen as the future of health care practice?
3. How is Monopsony a possible crime?
4. How can a prevention and education program reduce future health care costs?
5. What lessons have you learned from Hurricane Katrina that applies to health care providers?

Personal Observations:

1. Interview a professor or college dean in graduate school asking him or her how they see the future of graduate programs changing, especially how health care trends may affect their curriculums.
2. Interview five neighbors who are older then you and ask them what they think of the current health care system.
3. Look on the Internet for a Health Care Reform Committee in your state. Contact them, if there is a contact number or e-mail address, and ask for clarification of their purpose and their goals.
4. What is your belief? Should health care be a right of each citizen?
5. Interview a medical biller and ask his or her opinion about

being required to obtain a certification and purchase some type of bond or malpractice insurance.

References

1. Hogan, Michael, Health Affairs, September 9, 2003, An Interview With Don McCanne, M.D., "Why Incremental Reforms Will Not Solve the Health Care Crisis," **The Journal of the American Board of Family Practice**, May-June 2003, p. 443.

2. Ibid, p. 444

3. Ibid.

4. Don McCanne, "Why Incremental Reforms Will Not Solve the Health Care Crisis," **The Journal of the American Board of Family Practice**, May-June 2003, p. 1

5. "Health plans and hospitals join forces to address worsening health trends, "**Public Health**, Seattle and King County, www. metrokc.gov/health/news, May 17, 2002.

6. Crossen, Francis J., "The Delivery System Matters", **Health Affairs**, Volume 24, Number 6, November/December 2005, p.1544; also see **Crossing the Quality Chasm: A New Health System for the Twenty-first Century**, IOM, Washington: National Academies Press, 2001.

7. Shorftell, Stephen M., An Interview With The Robert Wood Johnson Foundation, www.rwjf.org/newsroom, 8/24/2005, p. 1.

8. Ibid, p. 2.

9. Magee, Mike, "Cross-Sector Partnerships in Healthcare," **Health Politics**, August 2005, p. 1.

10. Ibid, p. 2.

11. Enthoven, Alain C., and Laura A. Tollen, Competition

In Health Care: It Takes Systems To Pursue Quality And Efficiency, Web Exclusives, A Supplement to **Health Affairs,** Vol. 24, Supplement 3, Project Hope, Bethesda, Maryland, p. W5-420.

12. Mattoo, Aaditya and Rathindran, Randeep, "How Health Insurance Inhibits Trade In Health Care,"**Health Affairs**, Vol. 23, Number 2, March-April, Project Hope, Bethesda, Maryland, 2006, pp. 358-367.

13. Pugh, Tony, "Medical care in U.S. uniformly mediocre" Knight Ridder, quoted in the San Jose (CA) Mercury News, March 16, 2006.

14. Michael E. Porter, Thomas A. Stewart, "Solving the Health Care Conundrum," Working Knowledge, Harvard Business Review, Harvard Business School, September 28, 2004, p. 1.

15. "Blueprint For Fair Share Health Care", Consumers Union, May 24, 1999, p. 1.

16. Ibid.

17. Osborne, David and Peter Hutchinson, The Price of Government, July 16, 2005 www.governing.com,

18. Dinell, David, "A Perfect Storm," August 16, 2004, www.bizjournals.com.

19. Gingrich, Newt, "Transform It, Not Reform It," Washington Post, March 2, 2005, www.washingtonpost.com

20. Silver, George, Health Care: Beyond Markets, Washington Post, November 11, 2004, www.kaisernetwork.org.

21. Ibid.

22. Rick Romano, www.gmtoday.com, July 13, 2005

23. *A Century Foundation Guide to the Issues,* www.tcf.org, pp. 9 - 11

24. Gordon, Colin, **Dead on Arrival, The Politics of Health Care**

in **Twentieth-Century America,** Princeton University Press, Princeton, NJ, 2003, p. 11.

25. *Wall Street Journal,* kaisernetwork.org, July 28, 2005

26. Alan Radke, Governing Magazine, August 2004, p. 1

27. **Health Professions Education, A Bridge to Quality**, 2003, p.1, The Institute of Medicine (IOM), this report was a sequel to their 2001 report **Crossing the Quality Chasm: A New Health System for the 21st Century**.

28. Hefler, Janel, "Health Care Forum," The Martha's Vineyard Times, August 21, 2005

29. Gordon, p. 41

30. Ibid, p. 298

31. David M. Cutler, **Your Money or Your Life**, (Oxford University Press, 2004, p.114.

32. Arnold S. Relman, "Restructuring the U.S. Health Care System, Issues In Science and Technology Online,", Summer 2003, www.issues.org/issues

About the Author

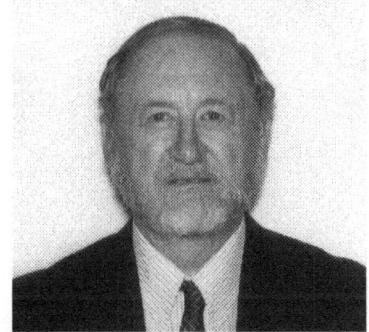

Ronald Hixson has been a therapist in the military and civilian communities over thirty years. He has an MBA from Webster University, MA in Psychology from the University of Northern Colorado, MA in Communication Studies from California State University, Sacramento, and a Ph.D. in Health Administration from Kennedy-Western University. He has been awarded the Diplomate of the American Psychotherapy Association. He has formed both a for-profit and non-profit mental health corporations in Texas, and he has developed a web site for providers and others interested in health care delivery issues: www.practicenews.com. He can be reached at ronaldhixson@yahoo.com. He is currently doing research for a second book which will explore the worth of health care services and how this can be used to promote parity in the general public as well as in the legislative halls.